Praise for

"Patient, nutritionist, educator, and author, Margaret Weiss takes the reader through the process of her experiences in the diagnosis of celiac disease, and in doing so, provides a roadmap for others. Graduating to nutritionist and educator furthers her insight into patients' experiences. This book is a valuable guide to being at ease with a diagnosis of celiac disease."

—Peter HR Green MD
Phyllis and Ivan Seidenberg Professor of
Medicine, Director of the Celiac Disease
Center, Columbia University Medical Center

"*Eat Your Rice Cakes* empowers both patients and providers alike to approach a major lifestyle change with not only objective fact but compassion for the very real humans involved in the process. With tips on how to establish a treatment plan based on the individual patient's unique circumstances, strategies for dealing with the mental and emotional toll of transitioning to a new lifestyle, and straightforward examples to illustrate any technique she mentions, Weiss has created something that anyone struggling with major life changes, not just patients diagnosed with chronic diseases, can benefit from reading."

—Alice Bast, CEO, Beyond CeliacBeyondCeliac.org

"Written with wisdom and heart, and a nod to the dreaded rice cake, Margaret Weiss has written the perfect primer for the newly diagnosed celiac."

—Jax Peters Lowell, Food Activist and Author of *Against The Grain, The Gluten-Free Bible,* and *The Gluten-Free Revolution,* an American Library Association Top 10 Food Book.

"Written for patients and healthcare providers, Margaret Weiss's personable health text, *Eat Your Rice Cakes,* forwards concrete advice about adherence, rather than compliance, to medical regimens. The tone is friendly, inclusive, and informative...

This is a book that can help patients and providers make the most of their relationships, and that can ensure meaningful communication and effective patient education. *Eat Your Rice Cakes* is a practical health text that will be useful when it comes to identifying stumbling blocks to medical change."

—*Foreword* Clarion Reviews
Clarion Rating: 4 out of 5

"In *Eat Your Rice Cakes*, Margaret Weiss melds her personal journey with her background in science to create the perfect handbook to guide someone through a diagnosis that requires a major dietary lifestyle change. With insight, warmth, and humor, the author embraces patients where they are, allowing room for individuality, grief, affirmation, and the vision to reframe and transform their future. This book—filled with compassion, clinical experience, and technical wisdom—should be required reading for medical doctors and students alike!"

—Ann Campanella, author of *Celiac Mom: One family's gluten-free journey after a daughter's diagnosis,* Director of AlzAuthors, www.anncampanella.com

"This is a warm, immersive book that comforts and clarifies with relatable descriptions of, for example, what it feels like to give up the 'moist and spongy consistencies of breads.' Weiss seamlessly shifts between her two intended audiences—patients and healthcare providers— while inadvertently appealing to a third: those trying to understand their suffering loved ones.

Overall, the author easily achieves her goal of shedding light on the emotional side of working toward a new normal, offering patients plenty of useful information."

—BlueInk Review

EAT YOUR RICE CAKES

DISCOVERING
EMPOWERMENT
AFTER A
LIFE-CHANGING
DIAGNOSIS

MARGARET WEISS, RD, CDCES

Eat Your Rice Cakes: Discovering Empowerment After a Life-Changing Diagnosis
Published by Wishbone Media, LLC
Frisco, Colorado

Cover and interior design by Victoria Wolf,
wolfdesignandmarketing.com

Names: Weiss, Margaret, 1961-, author.
Title: Eat your rice cakes : discovering empowerment after a life-changing diagnosis / Margaret Weiss, RD, CDCES.
Description: Frisco, CO: Wishbone Media llc., 2021.
Identifiers: ISBN: 978-0-578-79629-1
Subjects: LCSH Weiss, Margaret--Health. | Celiac disease--Patients--United States--Biography. | Celiac disease--Diet therapy. | Gluten-free diet. | Self-empowerment. | BISAC HEALTH & FITNESS / Diseases / Gastrointestinal | BIOGRAPHY & AUTOBIOGRAPHY / Personal Memoirs
Classification: LCC RC862.C44 .W45 2021 | DDC 616.3/99--dc23

Wishbone
MEDIA

For my wonderful and precious sons,
Dan and Tom, my favorite and most-often-used
quote (much to their chagrin):

"The biggest room in the world is the room
for improvement." ~Helmut Schmidt

And for the rest of my family and friends,
my second-favorite quote:

". . . they say you die twice. One time when
you stop breathing and a second time, a bit
later on, when somebody says your name
for the last time." ~Banksy

CONTENTS

INTRODUCTION

There I was with the door locked, cocooned in the tiny space of my main floor powder room, on full alert for unwanted observers. I had grabbed an entire unopened sleeve of Oreo cookies from our family snack closet and was systematically chewing and then spitting each cookie into the toilet, one after the other, without swallowing. Never one to dunk an Oreo in milk or split one open to scrape the filling off with my teeth, I popped each cookie into my mouth, whole and dry, just the way I like them. They tasted exactly how I remembered, chocolatey and sweet.

This was how I ushered in the spring of 1995, about four months after I was diagnosed with celiac disease. I not only had to learn a new diet that excluded a mysterious new vocabulary word, "gluten," but I also had to retool many logistics in my life, such as cooking, shopping, and traveling. My favorite warm weather activities, such as flower plantings, pool openings, barbecues, and kids' team sporting events, were unfortunately taking a back seat to the time and effort I needed to make these new adjustments. Happy with and accustomed to the varied, spontaneous lifestyle and eating habits I already had, I was a reluctant student. Reluctant to disrupt what had been working year after year, and reluctant to introduce into the mix what looked like difficult and unexpected struggles. I was the only one in my immediate family going through this transition, and the unhappy feeling that I'd had a "monkey wrench" thrown into my life put me in danger of spiraling into a bad place.

I really did spiral down that afternoon, cloistered in the bathroom with the Oreos. Having promised to start their homework after dinner, my two young sons were huddled in the basement, laughing and shouting as they tried to conquer the latest video game. Their father was not due home from work for hours, and I was alone. Alone and hungry. None of the food I had purchased for my new diet seemed appealing, and I was incredibly tempted by the smell of all those now-forbidden, gluten-containing breads, pastas, cookies, and cakes that were in the house.

How I loved those smells! The memory of eating those old favorites was still fresh in my mind. The familiar smooth and creamy textures of baked goods and the moist and spongy consistencies of breads were nothing at all like the crumbly, dry "imitation" versions I was now forced to substitute for my all-time favorites. I hated the changes I saw in front of me and how they clashed with how I really wanted to live. The habits and patterns that used to be enjoyable and easy were becoming unpleasant and burdened with lots of rules and restrictions.

Things change all the time . . . isn't our world evolving at what feels like a crazy pace? Many of us find ourselves with little choice but to greet changes to our personal circumstances in the name of progress and growth. Our ability to adapt to change is one of those unavoidable yet invaluable skills that are necessary to live on this planet.

But change also tends to shine a stark spotlight on its alter ego: the things that stay the same. When the dueling pair of change and sameness presents itself, we can't help but measure and compare the two. This juxtaposition is a lightning rod for our emotions when we stretch into a new direction or trajectory as we navigate back and forth between familiar comfort and unwelcome upheaval. And it's also logical that in this atmosphere, we cling a bit more to that familiar comfort. I know I do!

On that day in 1995, I didn't want to focus on the change that came with my diagnosis. In fact, my head was somewhere else entirely. I was absorbed with one of those favorite, familiar constants: the transition from winter to spring in central New Jersey.

Born and raised on the East Coast, I could always count on the predictable lush flourish that came after the gray winter typical in this part of the country. Just like a birthday or anniversary, I was celebrating the blooming of daffodils and forsythia common to where I lived. I also loved to keep an eye on fresh sprouts as they gradually appeared on branches in the woods behind our house, savoring my own made-up game of predicting the exact day they would—by some amazing unseen cue—all bloom at once and turn winter's bare trees and bushes green for the summer. Plus, I can't forget the predictable appearance of two robin red breasts that I swore to anyone who would listen were the same faithful pair that returned every spring to nest and feed in our back yard. These were happy events—predictable and enjoyable—and I looked forward to them every year. Yet, the spirit of my devoted ode to spring had been broken by the inescapable and unwelcome adjustments brought on by a change in my health.

Did my moment of sheer recklessness and defiance make me feel better? Actually, no it did not. Once I finished chewing and spitting out the cookies, I realized that I had added yet another element to the emotions I was already feeling: guilt! Guilt that took over most of my brain in the moment, leaving me to feel ugly and a bit evil. I had foolishly hoped that my spitting out the cookies after chewing them would remain undetected and do no harm to my body. However, the entire episode did nothing but demonstrate in very stark terms an overview of what was to be my new normal: initially, a desire for forbidden foods, then the internal fight of "should I or shouldn't I?" and finally, the resulting guilt if I gave in to my temptation and was personally responsible for hurting my own body.

I clearly grasped all of what my diagnosis and dietary changes meant to my health and everyday activities, and it made me feel even worse. I ached for the life I had when I could easily share meals with my family, friends, and colleagues without worrying about ingredient lists or the risk of cross-contamination. Now that I had celiac disease, this free and easy life was taken away and replaced with changes that seemed difficult and, frankly, unfair. I was beginning what would be a long, firsthand education in what it means to feel deprived, to feel different, and to have the need to plan ahead. I was experiencing what it feels like to "fall off the wagon," and all of the guilt associated with that. And I was forced to master the reconstruction of parts of my everyday life that would help me stay on my new regimen.

What a moment in time this diagnosis presented! Nothing would ever be the same. Life was no longer just about freedom and spontaneity. It was now about restriction, precaution, and vigilance too.

Many years later, I ended my stint as a stay-at-home mom, went back to school, and began a new and varied career as a registered dietitian and a diabetes care and education specialist. Now with about fifteen years of counseling individuals behind me, I have served in many different institutions and settings. I worked in the ICU for a large teaching hospital, wrote online articles for a supermarket chain, and counseled patients privately. A large healthcare system in New Jersey gave me the opportunity to start and manage a dedicated center that promoted advocacy, treatment, and education for individuals living with celiac disease. And, most recently, I spent several years as an educator for a major pharmaceutical company, providing diabetes education and training for physicians, office staff, and patients.

In all of these roles, one common element always stood out. No matter where I worked or what clinical prescription or diagnosis I was supporting, I had to promote new lifestyle changes to achieve optimal health. And these changes were usually drastic and required quite a bit of counseling and follow-up with my patients, whether they were managing celiac disease, obesity, heart disease, diabetes, or any other significant diagnosis. I could not help but tap into everything I had personally learned about change and my own forced transition as a patient with celiac disease, and apply the learnings to my work. I actually felt fortunate that I had had these experiences myself and could connect with patients about their own monumental life changes in such an intimate and sympathetic way. I know my patients felt that connection with me and welcomed it too!

Early on in my career, I came to fully appreciate the power that being both a patient and a provider can provide. One of my first patients, an eight-year-old girl, had sadly lost her beloved dog within days of finding out she had celiac disease, doubling her feelings of loss and disorientation. I confessed to her that I had lost my own dog a few months earlier and pointed to her picture on my desk. I could see the wheels turning in her head, and she actually said to me, "You mean you have celiac disease *and* your dog died?" She visibly relaxed, and we then used that picture as a launching pad to explore some of her feelings and allow for some much-needed commiseration and compassion. It was a perfect example of how shared personal experience can be extremely helpful when talking with someone about adversity. Since then, I have been continually impressed with how the mutual understanding that comes from a common experience results in better clinical improvement and faster emotional acceptance for the individuals with whom I have worked.

The array of challenges and opportunities both patients and clinicians face are many and complex, and the experiences and insight I have gained in both of these roles inspired me to write *Eat Your Rice Cakes*. Patients and providers each strive to manage change and achieve optimal health by conforming adjustments and new situations to existing lives and activities—although they reach these goals in different ways. I've seen a lot of what motivates and what burdens each of these two groups as well. How we treat change can be subjective, such as our emotions and feelings, or it can be objective, such as the information we find in clinical literature and textbooks. Rather than espousing or applying them individually, I've come to know that an approach that *combines* details from both "life" and "textbook" provides the best support to treat patients undergoing change. Because of this, I now embrace a blend of approaches to treatment derived not only from my own history but also from those of the patients and providers with whom I have connected and collaborated over time.

This dual perspective has historically opened the door to an incredible number of positive encounters, substantial growth, and sustainable healing for all involved. Taking this success into account, I wrote *Eat Your Rice Cakes* thinking initially about the healthcare providers—those dedicated, educated professionals who administer health-related treatment and advice to patients everywhere, every day. Providers, I invite you to explore this journey of change through my eyes. I know so well the wide spectrum of events, starting with the early, emotional struggles that come with the need to forge a new direction and ending with real-life, time-tested prescriptions for change. You'll receive an inside look into the patient experience that you may not have considered or appreciated before.

I've included plenty of helpful data and clues in these pages that will support your own journey to guide and advise others through different experiences, medical conditions, and clinical prescriptions.

I, myself, am always looking for new ways to enhance my counseling chops with alternate language, questioning techniques, or supporting data, and I actively "borrow" from peers, speakers, and presentations. Providers, your crucial role gives you far-reaching powers to execute immediate, meaningful change for your patients. The stories and encounters that I relate, both personal and professional, offer an inside view that can certainly help toward that end.

But I can't forget about the patients—I've been there too! Patients, it can feel overwhelming as you navigate change and new territory, and it's easy to wonder, "How am I ever going to manage this?" You may have happened upon this book on your own, or you may have been asked to read it by your healthcare provider. No matter how you got here, know that *you* are the ultimate benefactor of the work we do to help with understanding change and transition. For you, this book will offer important affirmations for your feelings and experiences. Plus, even though much of the information is geared toward providers and may get a bit technical at times, you may appreciate having the opportunity to learn different theoretical approaches to clinical treatment and get ideas about what you might look for and expect from your current or future providers.

Change. Transition. Adherence that is uncomfortable but necessary. What exactly do these concepts mean? And what exactly is the process to handle the disruption characteristic of this kind of change? Significant life changes take us on a journey of personal transformation, starting with an initial vulnerability and extending all the way to feeling capable and confident after mastering these changes over time. Once we understand change and our response to it, what then helps adherence and what hinders it? It all comes down to the ultimate goal of acceptance that takes place in our minds and bodies when the need arises. Our efforts would be well-purposed toward coming to an understanding, not only regarding how we process these concepts internally, but also what helps us move forward in the outside world and what tools will help us adapt and continue on the right path.

It's quite an undertaking, this change business. Just that single scene of my "Oreo Escapade," with its elements of concealment, longing, and guilt, underscores how hard and complicated change can be. Understanding this process is intricate and can also feel difficult, as life's circumstances are continually changing, frequently conflicting, and multifaceted. But never say never! I have seen and experienced success and opportunity more often than not. The journey is not easy, but there are many rewards and possibilities that significant change can bring.

Eat Your Rice Cakes builds on the ideas of change, transition, and acceptance, and suggests a way to navigate it all from a dual perspective. Yet, it's not a textbook. There are plenty of textbooks and technical resources available for patients and providers to turn to, but here we will spend more time acknowledging and incorporating the emotional side of diagnosis and treatment.

Curiously, this less clinical perspective is rarely addressed, although it seems perfectly clear how much our internal reactions impact our decision-making and behavior. From the perspective I've gained, I offer ways to understand why changes make us feel the way we do, with possible actions to take that are different from simple, traditional prescriptions of medication. In the following pages, I introduce ways to help cope with the negative feelings associated with discomfort and, most importantly, demonstrate forward-looking ways that are productive and healing to apply and cope with transitions and adjustments.

That forward-looking perspective then gives us the ultimate payoff: empowerment. Any life-altering change prompts questions about our place in the world and how to manage it. It is what we *do* with our experiences, how we ultimately emerge from life's curveballs, that is important to our story going forward. Change can be quite a blow and, as a result, we need to figure out how to regain our health, composure, and sense of self. Our reactions don't have to take us on a negative or destructive path, but can instead give us the ammunition to take charge of our lives and to rise up to new and improved opportunities and directions. We need learnings to build us up and to give us resources and inner strengths that steer us away from feeling vulnerable and victimized. This is how we find the power to heal and move forward.

The first gastroenterologist I saw after being diagnosed with celiac disease unwittingly delivered this kind of directive for forward-looking healing, although I don't think he realized or meant to do what he did, and it sure didn't feel helpful at the time. At that time, awareness about celiac disease and its only known treatment, the gluten-free diet, was virtually nonexistent. This doctor came right out and said that I was his first celiac patient and that, ha-ha, he vaguely remembered a chapter referring to it in medical school.

As for the gluten-free diet, he clearly had no knowledge of nor experience with it, either in process or in substance. Despite his admitted weakness, and without any understanding of the enormity of what he was asking of me, he delivered what he thought was an uproariously funny joke, something so unforgettable that it was the impetus for writing about my personal and professional journey: "You'll be fine, just shut up and eat your rice cakes!" I laughed outwardly along with him, but inside found no humor in the joke or comfort from his manner. The implication, of course, was that rice cakes are probably the least desirable food on the planet, but eating them anyway was—literally—going to be invaluable toward the overall goal of healing and health in my body.

We can look at the sentiment of eating rice cakes "for the greater good" in the figurative sense as well; life changes require incorporating into our lives any number of new and perhaps undesirable thoughts and actions that ultimately are needed to cultivate promotion and healing. It is actually a mandate to each of us when life is drastically altered: first, explore the challenges of change, then learn to "eat" or embrace life's adjustments on your way to healing and mastery.

I have carried the metaphor of the command to "eat your rice cakes" throughout this book, and we'll see that it works well not only with celiac disease but with all sorts of different medical situations and major life changes, such as diabetes, heart disease, and weight management.

To that end, we will first walk through the bundle of internal reactions I and others experienced when change is introduced: at diagnosis, via emotional expression, through the grief experience, and as a result of a path to accepting change that is frequently called "buy-in." Then, we will examine how established psychological behavioral theories and applications offer clinical guidance and reliable support for why we behave the way we do. Finally, we will explore how to put it all together into action that honors our needs, expectations, and environment. It's a combination of the subjective and the objective—an invaluable perspective for handling change.

At the end of each chapter, you will find specific concepts, or "Essential Highlights." Yes, a lot of the information in this book is meant for providers, but I invite every reader to examine this information to reinforce specific ideas and bring helpful input to the table, whether you are confronted with a brand new regimen or have been managing one for a while. We all want to mitigate our own discomfort, but I believe we also have a strong desire to inspire and bring joy to others, cultivate and enhance relationships, and apply new strategies to our interactions. No matter where you find yourself, I invite you to consider elements of this book that portray how counseling and treatment can occur in practical and humane ways, with approaches that allow development and rebuilding no matter what cards life deals us. By coming to know how "rice cakes" were managed in my personal and professional adventures, you may see patterns and similarities that aren't meant to promote a "woe-is-me" attitude but can instead be useful and provide insight into your journey. What has occurred in my personal and professional life is a portal to this bigger story of transformation as a result of change that I believe will resonate with readers from any perspective.

CHAPTER 1

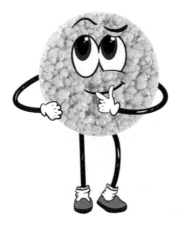

INTRODUCTION
TO RICE CAKES

Left on my own to "eat my rice cakes," I tried to make my way in this strange, new world. That was when I literally grabbed the lifeline that was thrown to me by one of the earliest gluten-free food companies.

Based on a mailing list I had somehow found and joined, I was invited to a food tasting to try out some of the new gluten-free items that this brand-new company was developing. The food tasting was held in a dreary hotel room not too far from where I lived, and for about a dozen of us, samples were prepared on every available flat surface in portable microwaves and toaster ovens brought in for the occasion. I can imagine that this setting might sound a bit awkward, complete with its supply of paper plates and plastic silverware sitting on the room's nightstands. But it was in this New Jersey hotel room where I first found connection and commiseration, and a little relief for the anxiety I felt in my isolation. We talked, we tasted. The experience was a faint beacon of light shining through what was a black hole of information and support.

Many years later, at a national conference for dietitians, I ran into the owner of this now-famous company and greeted him. "Remember that hotel food tasting in New Jersey you held in 1995? Well, I was there!" I said. Clearly touched by this memory of his early days with a startup company, he thanked me for bringing him back to that moment in his career and underscoring how small events and gestures can provide salvation when people feel lost.

WHAT WAS I REALLY DEALING WITH?

Celiac disease is an autoimmune disease where the ingestion of certain grains (wheat, barley, and rye) leads to damage in the small intestine. The damage occurs specifically on what are known as villi—small, fingerlike projections in this part of the body that are responsible for absorbing the nutrients we eat. When villi are damaged, the food we eat can't be absorbed well or at all. Without absorption, many nutritional deficiencies can result, including but not limited to weight loss, muscle wasting, osteoporosis, anemia, infertility, neurological conditions, growth deficiencies, and other autoimmune diseases.

As stated by the organization Beyond Celiac

(beyondceliac.org) it is believed that one in 133 individuals worldwide have celiac disease. Because it is hereditary, there is also an increased risk for individuals who have a first-degree relative with the disease.

The only known treatment for celiac disease is the elimination of wheat, barley, and rye (the proteins they contain are collectively referred to as *gluten*) from the diet. That includes Oreos! In the absence of these three botanically related grains and their proteins, the previously damaged villi of individuals with celiac disease are able to heal, remaining healthy and functional as long as a gluten-free diet is followed.

THEN VERSUS NOW

In 1995, there weren't many options on the grocery shelves for individuals following a gluten-free diet, and people with celiac disease were mostly encouraged to eat "naturally gluten-free," i.e., meats, vegetables, potatoes, rice, eggs, and anything else that naturally occurs without those pesky, offending grains. Other than that, everything else was summed up with one directive: "If you don't know what's in it, don't eat it." My experience with new products being demonstrated in a hotel room, as described at the beginning of this chapter, was a good example of how "off the beaten path" many details of this new, gluten-free life would be.

Of course, these days we are aware of an abundance of "substitute" foods for people following a gluten-free diet to enjoy: gluten-free breads, pastas, cookies, pizza, and more. Even Nabisco, the company that makes Oreos, has now come out with a gluten-free version of this all-time favorite. Plus, a lot has been done over the years to improve the experience for anyone following a gluten-free diet; ingredient lists have become more user-friendly, restaurants are much more accommodating, and general awareness about the gluten-free diet continues to grow. But those of us with celiac disease are still involved in a lot of anticipatory planning and playing defense on a daily basis, no doubt about it.

HOW DID MY FAMILY AND I HANDLE IT?

My family's journey with celiac disease began with just one family member who exhibited many of the classic symptoms, but it took several years to find out the exact cause. It is well-recognized that individuals frequently don't know what is wrong with them for an average of six to ten years, as celiac disease can be mysterious and elusive in its presentation. Admittedly, knowledge and awareness have improved over time and so have many of these statistics, but back in 1995, it was the equivalent of the Wild West in terms of diagnosis and treatment.

Because of the known genetic component of the disease, my immediate family was then tested, and I was surprised to be the only other lucky one. (Later, as my family grew in size and added another generation, three other family members were eventually diagnosed.) The chronic GI distress I exhibited during my childhood was explained away, as I was thought of as the "nervous one," and I really never showed any other of the classic symptoms of weight loss, deficiencies, or growth issues. As a matter of fact, I had grown to be five feet six inches by the time I reached sixth grade, and as an adult, I bore two nine-pound babies! We'll never really know when the disease started to affect my body, and it was precisely this lack of symptoms that made my diagnosis more difficult to accept and consequently treat with a gluten-free diet. Who wouldn't ask, "I'm perfectly healthy, so why do I have to make these incredibly drastic changes?"

And drastic changes they were. Since my sons and their father did not have celiac disease, I made the choice not to convert my entire home to gluten-free living. In time, I learned that a patient's acceptance and adherence are significantly improved when the entire family adopts the diet—especially when a child is among the newly diagnosed—but at the time, I thought it best not to inflict this restriction needlessly on the rest of my family. That meant several key adjustments within our home had to be made: my food was kept in a separate cabinet, cross-contamination protocols had to be set and understood by all, and we had to modify how we traveled and chose restaurants. Most challenging of all, I had to handle non-gluten-free food all the time as I prepared daily meals and school lunches for my family.

I was also concerned with whether or not my sons, seven and four at the time, had celiac disease. Soon after my own test came back positive, I held my breath and had their blood tested; they were thankfully negative, even after the meal of pizza and donuts I fed them the night before. I know it sounds dramatic, but that Last Supper of almost solid gluten—with its sentiments of farewell and finality—showed just how much guilt and anxiety I had about passing celiac to my children. Afterward, I found a pediatric gastroenterologist who would monitor their growth by running the celiac antibody tests and weigh and measure them annually. A few years later, when the gene test for celiac became readily available, I found out that one son has the gene for celiac disease, and one does not. It is generally recognized that most people with celiac disease have one or both of two particular genes, so I now know that one son will never be affected in his lifetime, and one son needs to be watched and retested as the years go by or if symptoms start to occur.

HOW ABOUT OUTSIDE THE HOME?

Do you know how people with celiac disease, back in 1995, were able to tell if their food was gluten-free or not? Not easily, that's for certain. It was hard, and resources were scarce. An employee in our local health food store initially took pity on me and led me down each aisle in the store, pointing out safe choices. Additionally, I found one—only one—national support organization at the time that offered phone and online support. This organization produced an annual summary of products that they had researched and determined to be gluten-free. This information was delivered to my house via snail mail in a loose-leaf binder, and the pages of this binder were updated every year and sent to my home to replace the previous year's version.

Happy and relieved to rely on something civilized in this new, primitive world, I took the binder to the grocery store and specifically chose the brand names mentioned in it that had been confirmed to be "officially" gluten-free. Talk about a lack of spontaneity and feeling different! Grateful for any guidance, I kept my binder current and waited eagerly every year for my updates, always hopeful for new additions to the "list" that would expand my repertoire of available, safe foods.

Of course, these days we have many ways to research ingredients and brand names electronically, not to mention reaping the benefits from the very reliable tool in the FDA's 2013 gluten-free labeling rule that defined acceptable levels of gluten and resulted in simpler and more easily understood labeling requirements.

Things got even more difficult when I needed to leave my house. I had plenty of friends and relatives who simply refused to accept or accommodate my new diet—some even made fun of it. I am not sure whether it was a lack of information or a simple refusal to acknowledge the importance of my new diet, but the result was that I frequently had to bring my own food or settle for eating unsatisfying or incomplete meals at many social events and holiday gatherings.

On many occasions, I patiently explained to my hostesses some easy and cheap fixes for the most common pitfalls of this problem that would accommodate my new regimen, no matter what else was served. Because I couldn't eat wheat-containing crackers or bakery pastries, I thought a suggestion for keeping handy a bag of corn chips to serve with hors d'oeuvres or a container of ice cream for dessert was a pretty easy accommodation. But these requests were mostly met with uncomprehending stares or just plain silence, and some individuals pointedly refused to help. Others told me that my food looked "weird," as much of my shopping was done at a local Asian market where a lot of the choices were rice-based instead of the very American wheat-based foods found in traditional grocery stores.

Restrictions, lack of spontaneity, and sparse support became the cornerstones of my introduction to this new life. I could see the stark reality before me as my "new normal" played out each day, and what was clearly an emotional journey of change began to take noticeable shape. The symbolism of rice cakes— what they represented in terms of these new changes to my world—loomed large, and I wondered what my future would look like.

ESSENTIAL
HIGHLIGHTS

- Celiac disease is an autoimmune disease that results in damage to the absorptive structures in the small intestine when gluten (wheat, barley, rye) is ingested. The only known treatment is the removal of these grains from the diet, better known as the gluten-free diet.

- There are many obstacles to overcome when learning about the gluten-free diet, both in and out of the home.

- No matter what disease state or prescription you are dealing with, keep track of new medical developments, new products, and changes to labeling laws, since these are continually evolving.

CHAPTER 2

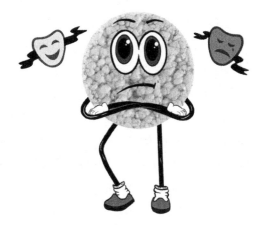

WHY DO RICE CAKES MAKE ME EMOTIONAL?

For about two years, I struggled with my new diet. Even though I didn't think I had ever exhibited any symptoms of celiac disease, with hindsight, I can see now that I did experience a range of GI symptoms, including diarrhea, cramps, and even noxious gas that I blamed on our family cat.

And, I can also now admit to an episode about a year after starting my new, gluten-free diet when I scarfed down an entire Irish soda bread while hidden in my car around St. Patrick's Day. With my sons safely at school, my travels took me near one of my favorite bakeries, and I simply could not resist the holiday display in its window. Temptation and guilt were at war inside of me, something that I immediately learned was an isolating phenomenon, since I didn't really have anyone to help me through this predicament. It felt like I was doing something illegal (what if somebody I knew saw me!), but I bought one of the breads anyway and returned to the car. Ripping off chunks of the bread piece by piece, I relished the taste and texture of each bite of that delicious, gluten-laden treat, and it was gone before I knew it!

During that time, I'd be able to stay on the diet a few months, and then life would get in the way: a party, a holiday, a bit of self-pity . . . and that's when I'd cheat.

It would be difficult to talk effectively about moving forward in one's change transition without acknowledging the initial emotions that we bring to the table when first confronted with change. Emotions are an important part of how to approach change! Whether you are counseling someone in this situation or experiencing this change yourself, this idea is fundamental. We need to recognize that emotions originate in our experiences, expectations, ethics, and everything else that makes up our individual life stories. Without a doubt, what we bring to a situation has a great impact on the solutions and recommendations that can be developed and implemented over time. Plus, a lot of the work we do to accommodate our emotions about change needs to be done within ourselves despite well-meaning input or guidance around us—it's not easy, and the process can be quite painful. I certainly can testify to this!

When I was diagnosed, I was really angry. Prior to my diagnosis, I didn't have any symptoms that I could put my finger on, and I felt great. Unprepared for the restriction and uncertainty of life with celiac disease, I had been living a life that was a happy, spontaneous jumble typical of a stay-at-home mom: meal preparation, grocery shopping, housekeeping, family activities, kids' activities, and caring for our dog and two cats, to name a few. It was only the protocol that all family members be screened after one family member tests positive that uncovered my own active disease. Just one sterile, objective recommendation forever altered my varied and carefree life! I remember literally saying the words, "If so-and-so hadn't been diagnosed, I wouldn't have to do this." I actually blamed my family member!

In the beginning, confusion and a sense of isolation weighed most heavily. Nobody knew enough back then to really be of much help, although I did understand that the implications for not mastering the diet and new lifestyle did not bode well for my health. It's quite a hard pill to swallow when you transition from complete command of your life to feeling completely at odds with your routine and general habits. And you can add insecurity to the mix, as I didn't quite yet have the confidence in my food choices that I would gain over time.

Back then, how could I not feel different? First, I had to lug that big binder with me on all food shopping trips so that I could be sure my choices were safe. Other shoppers had their coupon sorters or their children in the seat of the shopping cart, but not me. My big binder occupied that spot instead, its "gluten-free listing" and celiac logo loudly announcing its purpose to the world. It took forever to leaf through it, and there was no guarantee that I would find what I wanted or needed. Second, I couldn't always get my food in mainstream stores like everyone else could, but I had to make extra stops in health food stores and Asian markets. When I took my sons shopping with me, it was always a big joke about the characteristic "smell" of the health food store, and they held their noses, mimed gagging episodes, and provided many other preadolescent attempts to make fun of the situation. Then, when I finally got my shopping bags home, I had to handle and prepare non-gluten-free food and meals for my family since they still consumed a normal diet.

I was also particularly sad about my favorite food: pizza. It was incredibly challenging to find a satisfying substitute for traditional pizza crust, not to mention missing the spontaneity of popping into a pizzeria for a quick slice while shopping or traveling. I am embarrassed to say this loss was so great that, unless my sons were invited to a birthday party or other event hosted by someone else, I could not bring myself to buy them traditional pizza or take them to a traditional pizzeria during most of their childhood. Instead, we frequented some of our country's national pizza chains whose pizza was different enough from traditional pizza that I didn't feel quite so sad or deprived when seated at the same table, watching them consume it. Sad and selfish? Yes, but it helped to lessen my feelings of deprivation, and my sons didn't seem to mind. To this day, I offer a standing, substantial reward for acceptable gluten-free versions of my four most missed foods: pizza, Pop-Tarts, baklava, and spanakopita!

I also had to adjust to asking for special accommodations in restaurants and feeling frustrated when my needs or instructions were mocked, ignored, or misunderstood. Back in 1995, restaurants didn't carry gluten-free pasta (these days many do), but it was acceptable then to bring one's own gluten-free pasta and have the restaurant prepare it for you. I quickly learned, however, that restaurants save time and burner space in their kitchens by keeping a big pot of water boiling at all times, making pasta orders in it over and over again. Little did I know that when I asked the kitchen to cook my gluten-free pasta for the first time, they unceremoniously dumped it into this contaminated water and then served me my meal . . . and boy did I get sick!

Most annoying and frustrating of all was when I would ask for a hamburger without a bun, or eggs without toast, and had to listen to my waitress say, "Oh, are you on the Atkins diet?" Equally frustrating was my experience with a pizzeria that was a bit ahead of its time by serving pizza with gluten-free crusts. Unfortunately, they didn't really grasp the entire definition of gluten-free and included pieces of fried eggplant (fried with breadcrumbs) on my veggie pizza.

Without a doubt, I did have some positive discoveries, even though the breakthroughs they represented kept me on a roller coaster of emotions. I was lucky and thankful to find a bread machine that came with five excellent gluten-free bread recipes. The only downside: the loaf pan was circular in shape so all of my sandwiches were round, adding to the "food is weird" looks that I would get whenever I brown-bagged my lunches. More ups and downs continued with adapting holiday recipes for our multicultural family, as we developed original recipes for gluten-free *matzah* for Passover and gluten-free *zeppole* for Christmas. However, this took several years to perfect, and I spent many holidays looking wistfully at other people's plates at our family get-togethers.

It was a happy moment to discover that some spirits could be made from potatoes and other alternative grains, but these products were hard to find and were quite a bit more expensive than mainstream alcoholic beverages. Over time, the celiac community would accept that even if a product was distilled from a gluten-containing grain, the end product—or "distillate"—would not contain any gluten. This opened up a slew of previously forbidden items, such as distilled vinegars and spirits that made following a gluten-free diet in and out of the home exponentially easier.

Powerless? Paralyzed? Yup, I felt those too. I had to get all my medication from a special compounding pharmacy because back then, we weren't sure if drug companies used gluten-containing ingredients in their formulations. I had been the queen of finding sales and clipping coupons, but the changes I had to make took away the power I had over what and where I purchased, and the faith in whom I could trust. The general feeling of loss of control and the inability to move forward for fear of making a mistake overwhelmed me in my day-to-day activities. I had to rethink and retool almost every food-related project and process to make sure I could adhere to my diet, leaving my new life almost unrecognizable and heightening my sense of separation from the world I lived in and the people I lived with.

What a rush of emotions! Even a cursory look at this accounting of my experience is enough to give anyone pause. Isolation and anger, frustration and confusion, feelings of deprivation, loss of control, and, yes, envy. I felt all of these feelings but didn't know how to address them myself or with others. I was, after all, still a mom trying to keep up with the rest of our family's activities despite this new hurdle in my path. I buried a lot of my feelings and soldiered on, often disappointed or discouraged as I tried my best not to let my new restrictions interfere with anyone or anything else. Sometimes I was successful in overcoming these bad feelings, other times they got the better of me, and I felt sad, or I cheated on my diet.

These sentiments turned out to be initial stepping stones toward creating the acceptance and sense of purpose that would allow me to move on, a springboard from which I started to understand and incorporate figurative "rice cakes" into my life.

ESSENTIAL HIGHLIGHTS

- Change will evoke an emotional response. That response will depend on our past experiences, current expectations, ethics, and everything else that makes up our individual life stories.

- Emotions related to change can be strong. It's important to recognize and evaluate them because they can show us what may help or hinder our abilities to stick to a new regimen.

CHAPTER 3

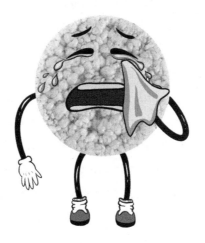

I'M SICK OF
RICE CAKES

Before I was diagnosed with celiac disease, I learned that I had another condition that was just as life-changing. Because of this diagnosis, I needed several abdominal surgeries over the next few years and learned that I would never be able to have more children. I had wanted one more for a total of three. For a very long time, I wrestled with how shattering my disappointment was and the fear of what the future would look like. I eventually broke down in tears during one appointment with the doctor who was treating me.

His response was, "Margaret, bad things happen to good people." I couldn't believe it, but with that one small sentence, it was as if two balloons had popped, and I immediately felt better. I could feel the pit in my stomach dwindle, and my face broke out into a small smile for the first time in a long while. That very compassionate sentiment accomplished two important things. First, it reminded me that I was a good person, that I hadn't done anything to deserve or cause what was happening to me. And second, it comforted me, telling me that this was indeed a bad thing, that the sad feelings I was experiencing were real and justified. In the aftermath of that conversation, I was able to take a deep breath and erase enough of the sadness and disappointment I'd been feeling to move on.

I've learned how common it is to hide how bad some things feel from the rest of the world and to blame one's self for adversity and misfortune. It's hard to find the inner strength to move forward when we feel this kind of mental distress. To this day, I use this doctor's sentiment when counseling my own patients, and I swear I can see the same relief and affirmation on their faces that I experienced so many years ago.

In that personal story, I was confronted with the need to make internal mental changes so that I could move forward and accept new changes in my body and in my life. I was disappointed and unhappy with what was occurring in my body, but I really had no choice in the matter and needed to find a way to manage my feelings so that I could continue living happily. This opening story and other life-altering changes that become necessary because of a dietary or medical diagnosis all have something in common: the result is giving up something we have wanted for the benefit of our overall health and longevity.

This contrast between a comfortable or desirable aspect of our lives and a new situation that may seem troublesome or unwanted sets us up to feel conflicted about how to react, how to proceed, and, ultimately, how to accept the change. To be honest, who really wants to experience this type of upheaval, disappointment, and extra work? An understanding of these very human feelings goes a long way toward the process of acceptance and empowerment—the ultimate goal in shaping effective change.

WHAT EXACTLY IS WORKING HERE?

It's common for us to struggle with the difference between what we want and what we need. These daily battles are frequent and varied, real and imagined. The classic image of an angel and devil, sitting on our shoulders and fighting over our decision-making process, has its roots in a poem written by the Roman Christian poet Prudentius, who lived in what is now northern Spain in late 300 A.D. His poem, *Psychomachia*, depicts the inner psychological conflict ("psyche") and the internal war between vices and virtues, wants and needs ("mache" in Greek). Here is an excerpt of his poem:

"Have you ever heard that voice of
reason whisper in your ear?
Oh, did it say the things you
never want to hear?
Tell me, where'd that angel perched
upon your shoulder go?
Did you pick her up and swallow her whole?
And do you ever miss the balance
of the back and forth
Or is it peaceful now without
the extra noise?
Tell me, where'd that devil perched
upon on your shoulder go?
Did it make your head its home?"

This poem describes the internal battle that begins with change. Whether you are a patient with a new health condition and a newly prescribed regimen, or you are a healthcare provider tasked with prescribing or describing new information that requires behavior and mental change, it is this conflict that must be considered as another impactful part of the experience.

There are tasks and activities in our lives that are fun, satisfying, and desirable on many fronts, and then there are those that are difficult and uncomfortable, but definitely necessary for our health and well-being. For example, activities such as dining out or participating in sports are certainly fun and desirable for most of us. However, a new diagnosis or life change can render any of these undertakings instantly unsuitable or unhealthy for any number of reasons, and this is where the battle between our wants and needs is introduced. For instance, soaking up the sun on the beach may be a much-loved activity, but if you take medication that causes sun sensitivity, you might have to either avoid the sun altogether or sit under an umbrella. You may not want either option but need to choose one in order to take proper care of yourself.

For sure, my personal battle described at the beginning of this chapter portrays this kind of inner debate as I wrestled with the difference between what I wanted (more children) and the changes in my body that necessitated life-saving surgery that prevented me from achieving my goal.

And why do we experience this battle in our minds, this seesaw of emotions that alternates between hailing our desires and facing our constraints?

Because I believe that during this battle we are experiencing grief.

Grief for what once was familiar, comfortable, and pleasurable. Grief for having to make an unwanted change. Grief for feeling forced into a future that looks unknown and, perhaps, even unsafe if the change includes serious disease or other physical or emotional challenges.

The now-famous five stages of grief, as promoted by Elisabeth Kubler-Ross, MD, in her book, *On Death and Dying*, are certainly applicable and appropriate as part of the objective and subjective combination best used to handle change. Here they are in all their glory:

- *Denial*: shock and disbelief that the loss has occurred
- *Anger*: that someone or something we love is no longer here
- *Bargaining*: all the what-ifs and regrets
- *Depression*: sadness from the loss
- *Acceptance*: acknowledging the reality of the loss

Grief comes in many different forms and packages. We typically think of the grief that we experience for a lost loved one as the most typical application for Kubler-Ross's famous stages. And I am, admittedly, not qualified or experienced to counsel about grief for a loved one. But I believe the stages of grief apply to any situation where there is a loss that must be acknowledged and accepted, such as the loss of a former lifestyle, a state of health, or a certain comfort level. The blow I received when I learned I could not have more children is a perfect example. It was a dream and a goal that needed to be acknowledged and grieved in the same way we grieve for the loss of a loved one. It was a vision that would never become a reality.

We can see this need to mourn loss as a result of life-altering change play out in many ways. Individuals newly diagnosed with celiac disease grieve for the foods and spontaneity they enjoyed before it was necessary to follow a gluten-free diet. People recovering from heart attacks frequently mourn for their former good health and lament the restrictive new regimen that is meant to preserve and extend life. Or, simply imagine how a new diabetic might wish for the simple, pain-free days before finger sticks and injections became the new normal.

All five stages can be applied to pretty much any loss in the human experience, not just the loss of a loved one. We *can* grieve for many different kinds of losses, and we *do*, whether or not we or anyone else acknowledges what is happening.

AND THERE IS MORE TO THIS STORY!

After collaborating with Kubler-Ross in further research about the five stages of grief, David Kessler, MD, went on to write *Finding Meaning: The Sixth Stage of Grief* and founded the website *Grief.com*. With these, he expanded on the idea of the five stages of grief by adding a sixth: *meaning*.

As grief after loss evolves over time, we spend a lot of time and effort reacting to and honoring our feelings. But eventually—and the timing of this evolution differs with each person—space in our brains opens up to include light after the darkness, comfort instead of pain. This is the definition of finding meaning: an explanation for our grief, a reason to keep going, a beautiful memory, or even a cause to adopt in honor of the loss. We can find meaning in many different ways, and it is this added stage that allows and provides for growth and healing. In *Finding Meaning*, Kessler describes this progression: "The grieving mind finds no hope after loss. But when ready to hope again, you will find it. . . . meaning matters, and meaning heals . . . healing doesn't mean the loss didn't happen. It means that it no longer controls us."

Indeed, the appearance of celiac disease in my life resulted in grief. The "Oreo Escapade" was a powerful expression and an almost textbook representation of how I wrestled with these stages of grief. I experienced denial and anger because I had not had any major symptoms as an adult and wasn't convinced I needed to be on a gluten-free diet. I bargained with myself to see what would happen if I cheated. And for a long time, I was angry and depressed, not fully adherent to the gluten-free diet until more than two years had passed after my diagnosis.

Meaning came when, years later, I became a dietitian and started a center for individuals with celiac disease, dedicated to advocacy, treatment, and education support—and I eventually expanded it to three locations in the state of New Jersey. Through my story, I was able to commiserate with patients about emotions and challenges associated with being diagnosed with celiac disease, and I shared details about what it took for me to ultimately accept and adhere to the gluten-free diet. In our support group meetings, patients identified strongly with my stories about my early difficulties with anger and my struggle to stay on the diet.

I also developed education materials to offer hints and tricks I had developed for myself to manage dining out and travel. And I consciously gave the type of logistical and emotional support I wished I'd had way back in 1995 but never got—even giving out my personal cell phone number so patients could call me from the grocery store as they shopped.

As time went on, it became clear to everyone that this kind of sharing of experiences and acquired knowledge bolsters positivity and acceptance for most people, including me! The opportunity at the celiac center to advocate and be a model for the celiac community was an honor and a privilege, and I am most proud to say that I acquired national recognition by peers and patients alike for this work. That was the very definition of those final stages in the grief process: acceptance and meaning!

All the grief in the world won't help us process our feelings unless that grief is acknowledged. Kessler called it *"witnessing"* someone's grief: "The way to help is to make sure that the person who is grieving knows that s/he does have your attention, that you are listening, that s/he is welcome to talk to you about her feelings." When this happens and is successful, we are better able to integrate these sad feelings into the process of change.

I've seen firsthand many expressions of "unwit-nessed" grief. Patients with newly diagnosed diabetes worry that they brought the disease on by consuming too much sugar. ("Is it because I binged on so much candy this past Halloween?"). Self-blame and mourning frequently come together, so thoughtful education can serve to "witness" this grief by replacing misplaced assumptions with facts. In my own story regarding my inability to have more children, my doctor gracefully witnessed my grief. He didn't say, "But you have two beautiful, healthy children already, so don't despair over this turn of events," as so many others did during this difficult time of my life. Instead, he recognized my feelings of loss and made me feel heard, which made all the difference as I made my way toward accepting this new situation.

Individuals can also experience what is called anticipatory grief. This is commonly exhibited as uncertainty about the future or one's well-being, and often shows up in the questions we ask and ponder. *Will I die? How can I get through the next wedding/ meeting/event with my new issue? How will I ever learn to like or live with this new food/regimen/status?* Our minds tend to race ahead as we think about what could happen, and there is a need to witness this unhappy recognition that the future might look very different from or scarier than what we imagined.

When the future looks different, we mourn or grieve for the past. We've seen so far that most people view change as "bad" because it is different from what they are used to or want; and they consequently mourn what these "bad" changes mean to them. Having gone through this myself with my celiac diagnosis and not being able to have more children, I have come to realize instead that the most reasonable way to look at this kind of change is that it is not "bad" but instead is simply "different." Thinking in this way, the perspective of "different" can become part of the acceptance process since it opens up possibilities for positive applications and forward movement. On the contrary, the "bad" viewpoint keeps us wishing for something that no longer exists, we can't have, or we may blame ourselves for.

Our concepts about what the future may look like revolve around preconceived beliefs we have about our world, even if they are not always based in fact. Imagine trying a gluten-free "knock-off" of a favorite cookie, expecting it to taste the same as the original, and then experiencing disappointment when it doesn't. Of course, it tastes different and feels disappointing— the new cookie is made of completely different ingredients! Logically, it's not realistic to expect that it would taste the same. Or, in the context of adopting a newly prescribed exercise regimen, the pattern or schedule of everyday life will inevitably change, and it's unreasonable to expect that the needed changes won't feel physically different, inconvenient, or uncomfortable.

One of my favorite ways to manage these expectations, because it is so easy and effective with both myself and with my patients, is what I call the "three times rule." With this, we consent to try a change—be it a new food, a behavior, or a thought—three times before we decide that the change is "bad." So for someone with celiac disease, experimentation with a new bread or a cookie or a pasta has to happen three times before that product is rejected (or given to the dog!). For someone with diabetes, it might take three tries with a needle to realize that it really doesn't hurt terribly or take too much away from other activities. My experience is that those who truly embrace this tactic are able to experience a much higher level of acceptance than those who give up after the first try.

My slogan of "not bad, just different" is another established tool to approach grief processing. It's called *reframing* our thoughts. Trying to erase, forget, or leave behind our hurt, loss, or disappointment does nothing more than discount our feelings and make us feel even worse. It goes back to Kessler's mandate to "witness" our grief, without which progress might not happen. How can we acknowledge and embrace our feelings about a "new normal" so that eventually we can move forward productively and happily? One way to accomplish this is by connecting to our loss by adopting fresh, nurturing ways of being or thinking. Reframing is a definite shift in perspective, a way to look at a situation from a different angle. Have you ever heard any of the following phrases that portray this kind of mental revision to promote acceptance? Certainly they are catchy, but they also help us understand that before healing can begin, we must identify or "name" what troubles us. I find that these phrases are an easy and quick way to steer and calm the mind so that problems can be identified and solved.

Name it to tame it.
Labeling reduces anxiety.
Name and reframe.

Oftentimes, people who are struggling with grief or depression are overwhelmed with negative thinking and have trouble balancing positive and negative thoughts and actions. In fact, a negative outlook can become repetitive or like a habit that needs to be broken. Reframing allows us to break this habit and allow more positivity to enter into our thoughts and actions. This happens differently from person to person. I'm sure you can think of different people in your sphere, some of whom deal well with adversity and some who have trouble managing in the face of trouble and may even succumb to it. Once taught the skill and benefit of naming and reframing, most individuals can move forward with the next steps in their healing process.

One example from my own "top ten" reframed ideas occurred during a conversation many years ago with an old friend. I was describing my interest in becoming a dietitian, which involved making time not only for several years of in-class education, but also for a year-long internship and a qualifying exam. The crux of the conversation revolved around the fact that I was still a stay-at-home mom, and it would take about five years to complete these requirements because I was only able to commit to a part-time schedule. I was forty at the time, and those five years to completion seemed endless and very far away. But my friend's comment changed my entire outlook: "Margaret, you'll be forty-five in five years, no matter what. You can be a dietitian at age forty-five or just forty-five." Boom, I was convinced! I constantly "borrow" examples from my own life in my efforts to counsel others, and this one really works to put another "angle" on a seemingly difficult problem.

I am a visual person. I love images—in pictures or in written and spoken words—that I can identify with, aspire to, or incorporate into my day-to-day life.

These kinds of images can be a way to reframe our thoughts. For example, I have been greatly inspired by the author Cheryl Strayed, who wrote *Wild* and *Tiny Beautiful Things: Advice on Love and Life from Dear Sugar*. In these inspirational accounts about tackling obstacles in very challenging situations, Strayed takes the reader on a journey in which many aspects of her personal life didn't work out or were disappointing. It is common for us to have an idea of what life "should" look like, even if it doesn't always turn out that way, and I found her way of working through, or "reframing," her grief so inspirational. It is exactly the kind of self-talk I engage in with myself and the kind of behavior that allows us to move toward acceptance and adapt to change in the face of adversity.

One memorable part of *Tiny Beautiful Things* is the way Strayed views unexpected life events. When life takes an undesirable turn and leaves our best-laid plans behind, she portrays that former life as a ghostly ship that has set sail without us. The ship symbolizes a life we wanted and perhaps cherished, but one that we can no longer live. Her best, healing option is to salute that phantom ship from the shoreline of our actual, present life. Here is the way she described it: "I'll never know, and neither will you, of the life you don't choose. We'll only know that whatever that sister life was, it was important and beautiful and not ours. It was the ghost ship that didn't carry us. There's nothing to do but salute it from the shore."

How perfectly this imagery fits with both my celiac diagnosis and the time I found out I couldn't have more children. There is the acknowledgment or *naming* of a changed life, the affirmation and *witnessing* that what was left behind was still important, and the good-humored way of hailing and *accepting* that missed life from a distance. After reading Strayed's book, I occasionally consider that sister life of eating gluten and having a larger family. Gazing upon my own "ghost ship" from the vantage point of my life today, I choose to salute it from the shore.

ESSENTIAL
HIGHLIGHTS

- Grief is a big part of the story of change. Acknowledge it yourself and look for others in your support system to take it into consideration as well.

- "Meaning" is an important part of healing, one that allows us to move forward with purpose or resolution.

- "Witnessing" allows the griever to feel heard and included in the healing process.

- "Reframing" allows an experience to be viewed and handled from a different, more positive perspective.

CHAPTER 4

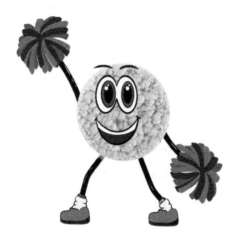

DO I EVEN LIKE
RICE CAKES?

Working in the celiac center, I once had an appointment with a boy who was ten years old and newly diagnosed with celiac disease. He came with both of his parents for the first installment of several educational and supportive "steps" I had created for new patients as they started to learn about this new regimen. In this initial meeting, I usually covered a review (age appropriate, of course) of how our bodies normally metabolize food, how celiac disease affects that process, and how to start a gluten-free diet. When they arrived, the boy practically slunk into the room, barely looking at me. From his monosyllabic responses and refusal to acknowledge the gluten-free goody bag that all new patients received, I could tell he was upset and angry. As I introduced myself and started talking, he only grudgingly listened to me, refusing to meet my eyes. He even blanched when I used the words "celiac disease" and said, "You mean I have a disease?" His mom, defending her son's distress, interrupted and asked me not to use the word "disease" any longer.

I'm sorry to say that as I continued with the education material, I eventually slipped—I was so used to saying celiac disease! When I made this mistake and said the dreaded word, the boy had clearly reached his limit and quite literally turned around in his seat, offering his back to me. Seeing his clenched fingers and the stiffness in his body, I didn't need to be an expert in body language to know that I had lost him. His parents looked at me wide-eyed, as if they had never seen their son act this way.

At that point, I knew I had to reel him back in. Talking to his back, I asked the boy if he played sports. He said that he was just starting football. I talked for a bit about how playing football was dependent on him being able to stay on the gluten-free diet so that he would get all the nutrition necessary to have and maintain the strength and endurance to play the game. Then I said, "You know, one of my sons played football when he was exactly your age. It was the hardest, most challenging thing he'd ever done, and he was incredibly proud of himself for enduring the pain, the grueling schedule, and the effort it took to maintain his grades in school during that season. He was so impressed with himself that he begged for a team football jacket to commemorate his achievement, even though it was quite expensive and not at all in our family's budget at the time. He wore that jacket as long as it fit on his body, and then when he grew out of it, he kept it hanging in his closet as a symbol and token of how hard he had worked and what he had achieved. He's a grown man now, and I think he still has it hanging in his closet. This kind of accomplishment can happen for you, too, and the gluten-free diet will help you get there."

Everything I said took place with this boy's back to me. When I finished, he turned around in his seat and said very softly, "OK, what do I have to do?" His parents, who had been sitting there taking in this scene, were completely astonished, with looks of combined surprise and relief on their faces. We then, all together, proceeded to talk about the intricacies of the gluten-free diet.

Months later, I bumped into this family in a grocery store, and I could see the mom pushing a cart full of gluten-free goodies, and the boy with a big smile on his face.

Buy-in is another mindset that adds to this multifaceted journey toward acceptance. Consider this quote by Chris Lytle that talks about how the simple act of promoting teamwork and acceptance in both players and managers tends to increase success with new plays on the basketball court. "You have to get buy-in as a leader, instead of demanding adherence to management. Phil Jackson sought Michael Jordan's support before installing the triangle offense."

We can strive for this type of partnership regarding health-related regimens as well. It's a pretty understandable sentiment: people need to find a way to appreciate and trust new ideas before adopting them. There is a big difference between actively "selling" a new idea or prospect for change versus thoughtfully creating a new vision by appealing to emotions, seeking feedback, and promoting compromise. There is a collaborative feel to "buy-in," where patients and providers both have a vested interest in the result.

It seems pretty obvious that my use of the word "disease" created a mental hurdle that prevented this young man from being able to buy in to this new change in his life, and I had to find a way for him to feel good about embracing this new journey. Making the connection of what he wanted (football) to what he needed (to follow a gluten-free diet) was the picture that I needed to paint in order to get his buy-in of his new lifestyle. Emphasizing the vocabulary and the disease simply didn't work for him, and switching gears toward more personal goals helped put him in the proper mindset to see what he needed to do. It sure helped to have had experiences with my own sons and other young patients to fall back on while counseling this young man—these are the compassionate and collaborative life skills that make all the difference in getting to buy-in.

It's similar to having a conversation; the first step is to speak the same language. Providers need to become part of someone's world through words or experiences in order to understand what makes him or her tick, what motivates him or her to change. Patients, it is so important that you find someone who will participate in this process with you. Successful buy-in lays the groundwork for progress, and it was with a special combination of gratitude and complete satisfaction that I saw this patient and his family out in public months later (HIPAA rules notwithstanding!), very clearly, appropriately, and happily accommodating the family's adjustments to his life change.

It is generally recognized in the healthcare community that creating "buy-in" related to medication adherence and other health-related regimens—like I created for my football-playing patient—is an ongoing challenge. And I've seen how both medication and food are equally difficult to manage when trying to improve health. The gluten-free diet basically uses "food as medicine" to treat celiac disease. Diabetes requires managing both diet and medication to achieve good blood sugar control. Weight management encompasses lifestyle changes that involve activity and diet. All involve some degree or combination of adherence with lifestyle or medication. So when it comes to creating buy-in, I think of and treat required food and medication adherence interchangeably because they similarly bring about a progression from initial discomfort to adaptation and finally to acceptance.

Regarding any regimen, there is a bit of divergence among us when it comes to the terminology related to buy-in. Some people talk about *compliance* while others use the word *adherence,* and this difference can influence success with buy-in. For a long time, patients viewed healthcare providers as experts rarely to be challenged. The focus was on treating the disease and focusing on generally accepted outcomes, not on the patient. Treatments, and those who provided them, were not expected to be challenged, and individual circumstances were rarely considered. In this environment, individuals were told to *comply* with and follow recommendations, basically deferring to the healthcare provider who occupied a position of authority.

More recently, healthcare approaches embrace a different perspective toward meeting the same outcomes; the needs and viewpoints of the patient are elevated in importance as compared to the simple focus on the goals of the healthcare provider. Patients are now viewed as *adhering* to regimens that are shaped by the inclusion of more individual involvement and personal responsibility. Patients in this collaborative scenario have the chance to provide input into how their treatment proceeds, more in accordance with their abilities, needs, and wants instead of solely those of their doctors. Patients are not dictating the course of their treatment, but they are certainly a greater part of the decision-making process than they were in the past. As I explain my attitude toward adherence to my weight management patients, "I could tell you to eat cantaloupe and cottage cheese to reduce calories and lose weight, but if you don't like cantaloupe or cottage cheese, what's the point?"

Additionally, the interactions that happen while working so closely together give the provider the opportunity to achieve greater insight into how the patient is managing their change and to predict his or her future behavior. For instance, finding the time or mental energy to shop for and prepare special food may require the patient to better manage time and have access to good information or resources in order to adhere to a new diet. Or taking medication at the right time might require scheduling changes or outside help with reminders. Perhaps on-the-job logistical arrangements need to be made so that a patient can inject insulin properly while working. And it's not infrequent that patients cannot afford the medication they need. All of these are crucial details that are quite significant and need to be incorporated into treatment plans. These details were ignored or rarely explored when providers demanded strict *compliance*.

An example of a provider living in the compliance camp rather than the adherence camp is what happened to me in what would be my last appointment with that first gastroenterologist, the one who joked about eating rice cakes. It was about two years after my diagnosis and we were discussing the recent holiday (Passover). I mentioned how much I missed *matzah*, one of the typical foods for this holiday, but that I had gotten through the event without straying off the diet. He said nothing and eventually wrapped up the exam. Then he gave me my chart and asked me to bring it to the reception desk (yes, this was before the advent of electronic medical records!).

Holding my chart, I peeked inside to read his note from that day's appointment. Who wouldn't?

He had written very clearly, "Patient non-compliant." Since I had *clearly* told him that I *hadn't* fallen off the wagon during the holiday, despite the temptation, I'm not sure how he came to think or write what he did, but I was extremely insulted and discouraged by his judgment and his refusal to explore this topic further with me. This had been a perfect opportunity for him to discover exactly how I was managing the fact that I missed *matzah* and perhaps to explore how I might find or make my own gluten-free version, or even to acknowledge that although not being able to eat *matzah* had been difficult, I'd refrained. Instead, I believe he jumped to the conclusion that I was lying about my eating behavior during the holiday and shut down any chance he had of engaging in meaningful dialogue with me, his patient. I'll never know if he misunderstood me or was simply disinterested in connecting with me, but this type of negative perspective about patients and a plain refusal to create a collaborative relationship makes it difficult to create buy-in. In my personal and professional experience, non-adherence is inevitably around the corner.

Soon after, I found another gastroenterologist to replace "Dr. Rice Cakes" (as I think of him to this day). The "compliant" imperative—that of blindly following a provider's guidelines without the benefit of buy-in—absolutely did not work for me. "Dr. Rice Cakes" had judged me without asking any questions or probing ways that might facilitate my adherence, even to the point of not believing what I told him. Contrast that to how I established common ground with the young patient about his chosen sport of football and steered our interaction toward topics with which he could identify and participate in. As patients, I think we owe it to ourselves to be treated with respect and compassion, and as providers I think we need to give patients the benefit of the doubt by not acting imperious, disbelieving, or requiring a cookie-cutter approach that doesn't fit with each patient's life.

I had another memorable experience with how critical and meaningful buy-in can be. In my role with a pharmaceutical company, I had a regular gig at one particular practice, a once-weekly diabetes education session that the doctor filled with patients on an as-needed basis. One week, as I was setting up our "classroom," the doctor approached me and said, "I only have two people for you this week. It's two brothers who live together, and their diabetes has been out of control for a very long time. I can't seem to get them to goal no matter what I do."

I started the class and casually chatted with the two gentlemen. They were in their mid-seventies, retired, and had been living together for many years. Their days were similar from one to the next and pretty much revolved around their meals: breakfast at home and lunch and/or dinner at one of those all-you-can-eat buffet restaurants that are so popular in certain parts of our country. If you are unfamiliar with this type of restaurant, they offer an extensive buffet and grill line. No grocery shopping or cooking for these guys; they had figured out that they could get anything they wanted at this restaurant without any work or planning. All they had to do was show up, make their way through the vast selection of entrees, side dishes, and desserts, and eat until they were full, all for a very reasonable flat price.

It was obvious to me that asking them to begin, now, to shop and cook for themselves was an unrealistic goal, probably almost impossible. And just as obvious was the fact that they were making choices at these meals that were not appropriate for managing their disease. They seemed attached, almost glued, to this lifestyle, without vision or desire for how to change it. So, the brothers and I started what would become a year-long conversation in the form of periodic "classes."

Every month or so, I met with them, coaching them on their choices at the buffet and comparing the accounting of their choices with their latest blood-work. We talked about the Healthy Plate model and how it could help control their diabetes. We talked about what their decision-making process looked like as they made their selections at the buffet and how choices from even this restaurant could be made to fit this model. As time went on and their trust in me grew, we were able to bat around ideas to gradually tweak their choices. I learned that I was the first diabetes counselor who hadn't told them to stop going to the buffet! And the tweaks were obviously working; over that year, they watched as their blood sugars went down, without changing a lifestyle that was clearly convenient and working for them. On top of that, their doctor was thrilled!

This was the very definition of creating buy-in: a collaborative process that included the desires of the provider (adherence with improvement in outcomes) and the desires and needs of the patient (in the case of the brothers, convenience and taste).

In my travels around this great country of ours, I think of these brothers every time I pass one of these all-you-can-eat restaurants. My memory of our inter-actions will always represent proof that changes are always possible, and those changes are easier and more fruitful when buy-in is created.

As you can see from my stories about the young football player and the brothers who frequented the buffet, patients can and should be given the opportunity to be open about information that, if given the chance, can aid in their care. And providers have to steel themselves against forcing information into the situation without first finding out as much as possible about the patient. When I worked as an educator for the pharmaceutical company, we had an applicable mantra: "Don't show up and throw up!" In other words, even if you come to a situation with your own agenda made up of preconceived ideas and judgments with wonderful and curative clinical recommendations, take the time to listen to and collaborate with your patients or audience before you speak and "throw up" all of that information in your head. This gives a much better opportunity to create buy-in and fit the "treatment" to the patient's personal circumstances and needs.

In addition, it's important to never underestimate the value that small successes have on your journey to get buy-in. As both patients and providers, we frequently have a preformed idea of what success is, but there are many versions and degrees of success. When looking for a place to start, creating trust is an attractive first step toward buy-in and success.

I once had a patient with ALS whose speech had so deteriorated that her caregivers felt a bit helpless to figure out how to make her comfortable, and she seemed resistant to new or different treatments every time they tried to help her. In our exam room, she kept saying the same thing over and over, but nobody could understand her. It was clear to me that she was extremely frustrated. After some very uncomfortable minutes, I finally grasped that she was trying to say "I'm thirsty!" Digging a bit deeper, I was able to determine that the family was quite conscientiously giving her food via tube feedings because she could no longer swallow, but had not realized that they needed to give her fluids through the tube as well. I was happy to help the family understand the "how to" and the "how much" education they needed, and the patient was far more comfortable and adherent during future appointments and procedures. Once she wasn't thirsty, she was more receptive to other interventions that could be added in the effort to improve her quality of life. Even though I had planned to implement any one of a whole list of *other* interventions on that day, I listened to her and stayed in the moment, ensuring that we understood *her* timetable according to *her* needs rather than mine. By gaining an understanding of her situation, I began to gain this patient's trust and we were able to implement other treatments that improved her quality of life during future appointments—the very definition of buy-in!

ESSENTIAL HIGHLIGHTS

- "Buy-in" is a crucial part of the journey to acceptance and adherence.

- "Compliance" is where the provider dictates the content and direction of a medical care plan.

- "Adherence" is where there is a collaborative attitude on the part of both the patient and the provider when creating a medical care plan.

CHAPTER 5

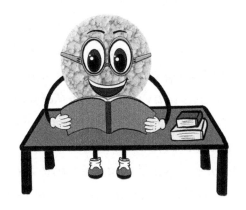

IT'S NOT JUST ABOUT RICE CAKES

One of my most discouraging encounters was when I was asked by a physician to counsel a patient with diabetes who was homeless and living in his car. With no room for storage or refrigeration, he was reliant on fast food for his nutrition. I sat with him and compared his budget with the menus at several fast-food restaurants to try to piece together some sort of diabetes-friendly regimen that he could follow in his unfortunate situation. This man freely expressed feelings of helplessness and frustration with his inability to stick to an effective regimen to support his diabetes and was clearly ashamed about his financial status and lack of resources that led him to this place. He also confided that he was afraid to take his insulin, as he had a frightening memory of an uncle who had diabetes and lost several toes soon after beginning his insulin regimen. It was encouraging, though, that this man was responsive, engaged, and willing to give anything a try. However, when the physician discovered that I had taken this unconventional route by helping the patient choose the best fast-food options that he could afford, rather than teach him a more formal and classic diet complete with fresh vegetables and low carb options, the physician was displeased and never asked for my services again. I am hopeful that this patient was successful in making headway with his disease and his situation, and I am also hopeful that this physician has had a chance to adopt more patient-friendly and productive approaches in the years since.

So far we've spent a good amount of time describing the emotional side of the journey from change to adherence, the first part of a combined subjective and objective approach to manage change. The second part of this combination, laid out in this chapter, relates to the technical and scientific side of things. Here we'll take into consideration some well-known models of behavior and psychological theories that offer actual data to support how our views of change affect adherence (or lack of it).

This objective information is the result of tests and research from labs around the world and is invaluable in providing other angles by which to view how behavior impacts our outcomes, our finances, and healthcare in general. Aside from the inevitable array of emotions my homeless patient in this chapter's opening story must have experienced, what other barriers were inhibiting his ability to stick to his regimen? What attitudes or preconceived notions might have been holding him back? The coming review of behavioral theories will shed additional light on these kinds of influences and will provide us with additional arrows in our quiver that can help to promote change.

My own journey would not have been complete without learning, understanding, and incorporating what I call these "technical" parts of the study of adherence. Whether you are a patient or a provider, observing behavior through this more objective lens surely uncovers meaningful ways we can manage change. For, as our former US Surgeon General Dr. C. Everett Koop so aptly remarked, "Drugs don't work in patients who don't take them," no matter what the reason.

WHAT DIFFERENT THEORIES HAVE BEEN DEVELOPED TO GAUGE ADHERENCE?

Behavior-Focused Models

Rosenstock's Health Belief Model
The Theory of Planned Behavior
The Necessity-Concerns Framework
Information-Motivation-Strategy Model

To start, some well-known models are listed in this figure, and you may have heard of them. These theories formally tested and now give clinical support to the idea that attitudes toward change and adherence have their roots in our personal experience and directly affect how we behave. To be clear, it is not the intention of this book to detail these behavioral theories at an advanced level. But even at a superficial level, their guidance has the ability to steer our actions, and learning about them adds invaluable insight toward our management and acceptance of change. Plus, I've also provided references in the appendix at the back of the book so that you can further research these theories as they apply to your own situation or career interests.

Consider the following:

- The models have documented the impact of how we view the seriousness of our situation or health problem, as balanced against the perceived benefit/barrier that adherence will offer.
- They have demonstrated that motivation and a sense of self-efficacy can dictate our behavior.
- They have uncovered impactful environmental cues (economic and cultural) that affect adherence.
- They have recognized cognitive development as a contributor to behavior.

These studies about psychological influences offer measurable clues about our behavior that are reliable and useful. To take just one as an example, Rosenstock's Health Belief Model examined the following variables for their impact on behavior and offered conclusions that we can use when we counsel ourselves or others about behavior change:

- Perceived susceptibility: one must admit vulnerability to disease first, before one can act to treat disease.

- Perceived severity: one must understand the severity of disease (and its consequences) before attempting to treat disease.

- Perceived benefits: one must believe that a particular treatment has the desired benefits before going ahead with the treatment.

- Sense of self-efficacy: one must have faith in one's own capability of treating disease before initiating that treatment.

You can see how just this one model measures what individuals value as they contemplate behavior related to improving health, guiding us in our work to improve adherence. Variables such as those listed in these bullet points are factors that we can work with! Patients or providers with this information can zero in on where to help improve perceptions and clarify information that might be holding back productive activity.

Boy, do I wish the doctor in this chapter's opening story had incorporated some of the guidance gained from Rosenstock's model when trying to help his homeless patient! Clearly, this patient did not think he could have a meaningful effect on his disease due to his homeless status (sense of self-efficacy). Plus, his memory of his uncle's experience with insulin, although inaccurate in the assumption that insulin therapy was the cause of amputations, was a definite factor in how he viewed insulin as a benefit (perceived benefits). From just this one model, we can see where a provider might focus in order to have the most success with changing behavior.

If you take a moment to read further about the other models I've included (find references in the appendix), you can see more variables that have been tested and shown to be impactful on our view of behavior. Or you can search the internet for what have been coined "technique demonstration videos," some of which show an actual therapy session in progress with subtitles that list the psychological theories and techniques being utilized by the provider during that session. No matter where you find it, this objective commentary and clinical support is an invaluable complement to what we know about the subjective body of our emotions.

Patient-Centered Models

Additionally, it is now generally accepted that a shift in patient interaction, called Patient-Centered Care (PCC), is another popular model that has significant value in addressing our reaction to change. The National Academy of Medicine, an independent arm of the National Academy of Sciences that provides objective, health-related opinions to the public, promoted PCC as one of its six formal objectives for healthcare in the twenty-first century. Specifically, the National Academy of Medicine defines PCC as "care that is empathic, compassionate, well-coordinated, and actively engages patients in decision-making." Thus, this model of care takes into consideration a person's individuality and employs that individual as a partner in their own care. Over time, studies have revealed measurable changes to adherence behavior when PCC is employed—both in the near and long terms and regarding overall patient satisfaction as well. It appears as if the National Academy of Medicine has created a formally recognized version of buy-in.

Any patient-centered counseling would take into consideration the homeless patient's situation, rather than force on him the traditional dietary models that his physician clung to. It's the very definition of a partnership, and it would serve both patients and providers well to keep this in mind in order to affect change.

Culture-Centered Models

Another formal theory that provides a slightly different angle by which to evaluate and influence adherence behavior revolves around the hypothesis that increased cultural competency of a provider leads to increased patient adherence. Cultural competency is a basic understanding and respect for people's skills, practices, and world views across cultures. This insight into diversity is a powerful force in promoting positive and productive interactions with people around the world.

In a 2013 study published by Somnath Saha, MD, MPH, et al. in the *Journal of General Internal Medicine*, providers from four outpatient facilities in the US were surveyed about four concepts: awareness of culture, how to relate patient care to sociocultural issues, social disparities within healthcare, and the consequences of different health behaviors and beliefs. The providers' answers were then compared to their own patients' outcomes and adherence. The researchers found that the more cultural competency the provider exhibited, the more the patient was adherent to his/her regimen. And the data showed the adherence was even higher in non-white patients. So, this study gives us clear, objective guidance on how to improve adherence *and* improve racial/ethnic disparities by simply increasing and expanding our knowledge of different cultures and practices.

This concept of the importance of cultural competency was certainly borne out for me at one particular diabetes support group meeting where I was asked to discuss portion control. The class happened to be entirely Hispanic, and they were struggling with how to manage their goals and my recommendations for carbohydrate consumption. I was happy to show some of my tried-and-true examples that I had successfully used for many years, one of which was my favorite example of how to portion out pasta, complete with visual aids. It was logical, practical, and visually help-ful. Many previous patients and classes had loved this example and vowed to use it in their own homes. This class, however, politely listened, and when I was done, someone timidly raised a hand and said, "But we don't eat pasta."

This group certainly drove home the fact that their participation, engagement, and any improvement in their overall health would be limited unless I improved and developed the cultural competency of my dietary counseling strategies. When I later did exactly that for them with a lesson about portioning the foods *they* ate on a regular basis, that positive relationship between the cultural competency of the provider and a patient's adherence kicked in, just like in the studies!

MODELS OF BARRIERS TO ADHERENCE

For sure, psychological theories like those detailed

earlier support the treatment of change by measuring how attitudes and beliefs affect behavior. But there are also other known challenges to adherence that can get in our way. Some of these challenges have been coined "barriers," and there are two types: concrete barriers and psychological barriers.

Concrete barriers are easily defined as being functional or logistical and are less abstract than psychological barriers. Lots of work has been done to examine both of these types of challenges to adherence, resulting in many proactive prescriptions for behavior change that lead to improvement in outcomes. Again, there is a general acknowledgment that these identified barriers don't only exist with medical therapies but can easily and effectively be applied to most lifestyle recommendations as well (such as weight management and exercise/activity levels).

Concrete Barriers

Executives in the drugstore chain Walgreens saw the need to specifically recognize and address concrete barriers to medication adherence—those logistical and strategic limitations that crop up in our normal day-to-day activities and get in the way of adherence. They hired over two hundred "health outcomes pharmacists" in March 2019, specifically to reach out to identified patients to try to uncover why they failed to refill prescriptions.

For those with transportation issues, these pharmacists enrolled the patients in Walgreens' delivery program or changed the order to a ninety-day prescription so that fewer trips to the pharmacy would be needed. If cost presented a problem, the pharmacists looked for lower-cost alternatives and worked with the patient's insurance company and provider's office to make that change. For many, it was also helpful for the pharmacist to arrange for "medication synchronization," where the patient could pick up multiple prescriptions at the same time. These tangible changes were quite effective, to the tune of an 8.7 percent higher refill rate in patients who had contact with these pharmacists, as opposed to those who did not experience this intervention at all.

Certainly, concrete barriers, by definition, are easier to identify and perhaps to address. As a dietitian, I've frequently helped with devising schedules, lists, or new ideas to help with the logistical aspects of new regimens. These kinds of barriers aren't really hard to understand or difficult to process; sometimes all that is needed is a pair of fresh eyes or the help of someone who has additional experience and resources to identify and fix the problem. It should be easy enough for a professional to guide someone with a new regimen, given a modicum of training and expertise. My work with the homeless diabetes patient included addressing concrete barriers that affected his situation, such as budgeting, lack of refrigeration, and finding handy, carb-counting aids for his car. And Dr. Koop was right—any one of these barriers, if left unaddressed, was capable of preventing this patient from taking his medication so that it would work.

Psychological Barriers

It is the psychological barriers that are more difficult to identify and manage. I'm not saying that concrete barriers are less impactful on overall health; their existence can, in fact, prevent health and healing in a big way. But the psychological barriers surrounding change create another challenge that is less clear and requires analysis in a more indirect way. These kinds of barriers are more challenging because they involve a complicated interaction between the individual, his/her personal history, and whoever or whatever is promoting a new or changed regimen. When we come up against a psychological barrier, it's because the personal history brought to any situation so greatly affects our actions.

To illustrate this idea of how our history might affect our present circumstances, I often think about when I was a beginning nutrition student, when my Nutrition 101 class focused on the role of food in our lives. "*Food* is everything" was the basic theme, since what we eat takes on so much importance to all of us in many different ways. Food is social, it is physically comforting, and its function in our lives has origins in religion, economics, where we live, and our personal history. We know that this background has a direct influence on future behavior in the face of change. Now, with years of nutrition counseling under my belt, I have adopted a direct translation of this sentiment and changed it to: "*Adherence* is everything." In other words, the act of adherence is influenced by past experiences and environments in the same way we are influenced by and view the foods in our life.

Thus, our ability to adhere to new regimens can take cues from our upbringing (emotional) and our environment (physical), and these cues can have significant positive and negative impacts on behavior related to adherence. If we think about the Asian patient with diabetes who must now adjust his/her consumption of rice, or if we consider how the ritual of Communion with gluten-containing wafers might be altered for someone with celiac disease, it is surely possible to see how the influence of culture, religion, and other parts of our background might cause some dissonance in the face of new change. When a former staple or cornerstone of our life is challenged by a new regimen, input from our background comes into play and can make adherence more difficult. This is really the definition of a psychological barrier.

I once saw an interview on a cooking show that illustrates this well. A woman, who had just survived a harrowing escape from her native North Korea and was now living safely in South Korea, admitted to some nostalgia for the North Korean foods and recipes she had grown up with and left behind.

Unbeknownst to her, the show's host had arranged for her favorite childhood recipe to be prepared. When she saw the dish, you could see how meaningful it was for her to experience eating this food after such a long exile. The TV world watched as she closely examined and touched the pieces, smelling them, tasting them, genuinely experiencing and connecting to her memories of eating this dish from earlier times. One could clearly see how eating this food conjured up lots of happy feelings and memories from her past.

> *"Food is everything we are. It's an extension of nationalist feeling, ethnic feeling, your personal history, your province, your region, your tribe, your grandma. It's inseparable from those from the get-go."*
> —Anthony Bourdain

However, I know the converse is also true: removing a much-loved or relied-upon staple that is so much a part of our history can result in feelings of deprivation and lead to non-adherence, even if that removal is considered life-saving. That is why I believe the sentiments "food is everything" and "adherence is everything" are interchangeable. The history we bring when we are tasked with life-altering change has a great effect on our future behavior, both positive and negative. Gaining knowledge of this history is invaluable in determining the best way to reinforce adherence and move productively forward.

WHAT ARE SOME EXAMPLES OF PSYCHOLOGICAL BARRIERS TO ADHERENCE?

We've all been there. Finding a new weight-loss diet so restrictive, and our hunger pangs so loud, that we quit after a few days. Or the side effects of a new medication are so unpleasant that we stop taking that medication or split the pills in half, just to feel better even if the desired medical effect is not achieved. Perhaps we get tired of or haven't completely accepted our new regimen and "take a break." These are examples of the psychological barrier called *intentional* non-adherence, and it is perfectly illustrated by the story I tell over and over again to my patients about the grandmother of one of my patients.

When I was running the celiac center, I had an elementary school-age child whose bloodwork never returned to normal after an initial diagnosis of celiac disease. (Bloodwork is done routinely for those with celiac disease to see if the antibodies that cause the intestinal damage characteristic of celiac disease are there or have returned. Most likely, if antibodies are found in the blood, then gluten is present in the diet.) After discussing this issue at great length with the mom, I gleaned the truth: the child's grandma, who was in charge of the child's care during the day, "didn't believe" in celiac disease and was "sneaking" gluten-containing foods to the child on a fairly regular basis. I never interviewed this woman, but wouldn't it have been interesting to uncover what was in her history that prevented her from positively supporting her grandson's new diet! Nonetheless, in this case, there were *intentional* barriers that needed to be overcome.

In contrast, there are other reasons we experience a psychological barrier where there is *unintentional* failure to adhere to something. We might forget to take a medication on time, despite setting an alarm or purchasing the "perfect" pill dispenser. We might attend a holiday dinner and reach for our favorite dish out of habit or forgetfulness, despite having a new diet restriction. Or, despite our best intentions, we might forget some of the instructions we received in the doctor's office and render a new regimen ineffective as a result.

The following quote applies a bit of humor to this idea that the burden of a new diagnosis and the new information that comes with it can be overwhelming. For this reason, I purposefully bring my husband to some of my more complicated doctor appointments, simply because he remembers details and instructions that I frequently don't recall. And, as a dietitian, I have become quite accustomed to the "deer-in-the-headlights" look when I describe new information to my patients.

Medical studies indicate most people suffer
a 68% hearing loss when naked.
—UnitedHealth Foundation

A woman who had just started injectable therapy for her diabetes showed me a perfect example of what it looks like to experience an unintentional psychological barrier. I was replenishing education materials in a back storage room at one of my biggest diabetes practices when one of the doctors came out of an exam room, saw me, and motioned for me to come to where he was standing in the hallway.

"I'm so glad you are here! I can't seem to get this patient's blood sugar under control. She seems to run even higher today than when I started her on insulin two weeks ago. Do you have time right now to talk to her? Maybe you can figure out what is happening."

Of course I would help. I went into the exam room and met a lovely woman, probably about sixty-five years of age. We chatted amicably for a bit, and then I asked her how it was going with her new insulin regimen.

"I thought it was going fine," she said, "and it didn't really hurt like I thought it would! But now I'm here, and the doctor isn't happy because my blood sugar isn't getting any better."

I explained that there is so much to get used to when starting insulin injections, and that I was there to help figure out if there was anything that could be adjusted. We reviewed her regimen; she fully knew what medicine to take and had her schedule down pat.

I asked, "Do you have your pen with you? Let's make sure everything is all right with that."

She nodded, reached into her pocketbook, and pulled out the insulin pen, still in its original box. But the box was dripping! Literally wet, the ink on the cardboard was blurry in some places and completely worn and gone in others. I could smell that characteristic smell of insulin, which smells sort of like Band-Aids.

"Why is the box wet? Did you drop it somewhere?" I asked.

"No," she said. "It got wet right after I started using it. I just thought it was supposed to be like this."

I examined the box and the pen. The pen seemed fine, just inexplicably wet. "Let's go over how you use the pen, just for a review," I said.

We reviewed how to inject insulin with the pen, and, lo and behold, she recited the entire process perfectly *except* she never removed the small inner cap before injecting. No wonder her blood sugar was not improving! All of her insulin doses were being injected into the cap and slowly leaking out all day into her pocketbook. And of course she experienced no pain, since the cap was covering the needle. Although I'm sure she had received hands-on training for injection therapy (including the removal of the inner cap on an injectable device), some of this instruction had clearly been forgotten.

New equipment, required behavioral changes, and new ways of doing a task can all feel overwhelming initially, leading to missed information and unintentional non-adherence. This can come into play for people with diabetes when they learn how to transition to injectable therapy after oral drugs have failed to control blood sugar adequately. As difficult as this stage is mentally and emotionally, added to the mix is the necessary proficiency with all of the "tools" and processes related to injections. First, the features of the equipment, such as caps, labels, expiration dates, and dosing calibration markings, must be learned. Then comes understanding the best location for injection, the timing, the cleansing with alcohol wipes, the priming of the device to ensure proper delivery of the medication, how to inject, and even how to dispose of the used equipment and accessories. Phew! All of that information and all of those details can be a perfect setup for failure, for unintentional non-adherence to sneak in. As an educator, I can tell you that it takes me at least an hour to disseminate all of this information, *and* ask the patient to "teach back" what has been learned so that I know at least enough information has been absorbed to begin treatment at home.

I must add, however, that current restraints on doctors and other providers, such as the time they are allowed to spend with each patient, can get in the way of the kind of exploration and empathy needed to uncover such individual adherence barriers, intentional or not. Truth be told, one of the last healthcare systems I had contact with when I worked for the pharmaceutical company mandated that doctors spend no more than twelve minutes with each patient. That's barely enough time to greet each other, commiserate about the weather, and ask, "What brings you here today?" I am always happy to make up this time for patients, as I was and still am able to "fudge" my time to allow extra minutes for some real detective work and problem resolution to stave off those pesky barriers as much as possible.

WHO IS NON-ADHERENT?

This section includes a good visual that shows some of the many reasons individuals are non-adherent with medication and health-related therapies. Is it possible to match the reasons for non-adherence depicted in this chart with some of the "technical" approaches we've just explored? Absolutely! Broadening our use of the Patient Centered Care model would sure go a long way if the patient doesn't feel needed or has a poor relationship with his/her physician. Uncovering and working through perceived intentional and non-intentional barriers can focus on affordability, forgetfulness, poor social support, or side effects. And understanding the behavioral models that explain how our history affects our actions sheds light on how to help patients who have low satisfaction with their medication, lack of concern with the diagnosis, or trouble processing information.

Reasons for Medication Non-Adherence

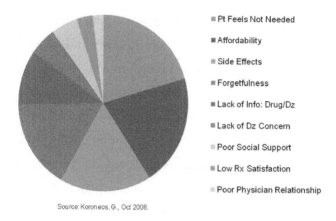

- Pt Feels Not Needed
- Affordability
- Side Effects
- Forgetfulness
- Lack of Info: Drug/Dz
- Lack of Dz Concern
- Poor Social Support
- Low Rx Satisfaction
- Poor Physician Relationship

Source: Koroneos, G., Oct 2008.

The technical guidance we get from established theory and studies is relevant and useful, and complements the role of emotions in the journey of change. It is clear that we are affected by both subjective and objective cues when we approach any situation, and Dr. Koop's fear that these obstacles inhibit adherence and healing is justified. Our lives and experiences are varied and complicated, and reasons for non-adherence come in just as many shapes and forms. I'm sure any one of us can think of even more variations, and there are solutions and prescriptions in the coming pages that are just as multifaceted.

NOW SOME STATISTICS: HOW MUCH IS THIS IDEA OF ADHERENCE WORTH?

Now that we have delved a bit into the subjective and objective components affecting adherence, it's also important to understand costs and benefits related to adherence. Why? If we can compare insight about our behavior with where money is being spent, where money is still needed, and how people's health outcomes are related to these spending and lifestyle behaviors, then we can better focus our efforts on shaping these expenditures and improving those outcomes. Because, of course, treating illness and improving outcomes are the ultimate goals, right? If we improve how we integrate all of this information, all the better ammunition to work with.

For example, think about what happens when we don't stick to our regimens due to non-adherence. People with diabetes who have trouble managing their diet and medication are frequently hospitalized for blood sugar that is too high or too low. Individuals who suffer a heart attack or other cardiovascular events are frequently readmitted to the hospital for the same or a related issue a short time later. Per the CDC, increased visits like these to the doctor, the hospital, or the ER all result in significant costs, to the tune of an estimated $290–300 billion per year. Then there are other significant and noteworthy costs that happen to us personally when we don't adhere to our regimens—these are paid not in dollars but in suffering and quality of life. No matter who we are, increased costs put us at a disadvantage within the healthcare system, in our wallets, and in our bodies. Clearly, non-adherence is a factor in that cost.

Contrast this with the considerable global spending on specific health-related diets that exist today. For example, researchers have determined that the value of just the gluten-free food market around the world was a bit shy of $22 billion in 2019 and is expected to grow at an annual rate of about 9 percent between 2020 and 2027. Quite a big number, and that doesn't even include food that supports any other food intolerances, allergies, or treatments!

Where non-adherence had a cost, one can see a general recognition that money spent on a particular diet to provide food for a particular regimen goes a long way toward adherence. Thinking back to when I started following a gluten-free diet in 1995, I remember basically one company that supplied all of the stores with rather inferior—albeit gluten-free—products. If the incredible variety and improved quality of gluten-free foods that are available today had been available to me back then, I think my feelings of deprivation might have been reduced and my initial efforts with adherence to the gluten-free diet might have been more successful. These days, when you see the grocery shelves overflowing with low-salt, low-fat, low-carb, and other nutritionally conscious products, we are reminded that these products are designed to enhance health and keep people out of the hospital by making adherence to health-related regimens easier and more enjoyable.

Statistics like these show us that expenditures and behavior geared toward increasing adherence can be impactful to patients and healthcare institutions alike. So impactful that the healthcare industry has developed targeted programs to identify and improve the health outcomes of specific groups of people (populations). Collectively known as Population Health Management, these initiatives track data about individuals within groups of people and use that aggregate data to improve clinical results and lower costs for both healthcare institutions and for the patient. It's where finance and clinical practice intersect!

These days, if you go to any physician's office, you will see the walls covered with bulletin boards or other public postings of how they are tracking lab results of individuals with specific health conditions in the practice—such as diabetes, hypertension, or heart disease—because programs like these have established that getting good, upfront control of these disease states in certain populations keeps a significant percentage of patients out of the hospital. This preventive stance works so well that insurance reimbursement and other methods of rating a physician's practice are tied to the tracking of these results, providing significant incentive for providers to engage with patients and their treatment in this way. The concept of Population Health Management thus guides healthcare providers in the comprehensive treatment of their patients according to the latest data and best practices available.

To come full circle, the data behind the theories in this chapter sheds lots of new light on how to counsel my patient in his homeless situation, despite the fact that his doctor did not embrace or choose to use any of this valuable information. For sure, the patient expressed a range of emotions that has now become familiar: frustration, a sense of isolation, and feelings of failure about not being able to maintain his regimen. But we can also examine his actions and attitudes through the lens of the formal psychological theories, offering help and counseling that his physician frankly missed.

We can ensure that the direction he receives is collaborative, according to the Patient Centered model, so that he can contribute ideas and suggestions about his budget, lifestyle, or anything else that might give insight into what would help him stick to his regimen. Or, a more culturally sensitive approach might address favorite foods or cultural rituals that are missing in his life and that would make him feel more comfortable and able to do what he needed to do.

We can also work with and shape his attitudes about his sense of self-efficacy, perceived benefits of adherence, and the perceived severity of his disease (elements of Rosenstock's model) now that we know how impactful his perceptions of these concepts are in the quest for positive growth and healing. These are all valuable opportunities, none of which would be included in the physician's cookie-cutter vision of a formal "diabetes" diet.

I very much appreciate these important, established models and theories that contribute to the way we consider behavior in order to help people ultimately gain positive outcomes. By understanding the way in which these models measure the connections between our inner perceptions and our subsequent reactions, we can help ourselves or others when confronted with change.

ESSENTIAL HIGHLIGHTS

- Behavioral models provide us with objective data that guide us in the treatment process. See the appendix for more references and resources about these models.

- PCC aligns a patient's needs and preferences with their medical care.

- Cultural competency defines an individual's ability to understand and interact with people and activities from other cultures around the world.

- Barriers to adherence impact behavior. Unintentional barriers are those that get in the way of adherence (financial constraints, forgetfulness, obstacles that prevent filling a prescription) and occur even though an individual really does want to adhere to a regimen. Intentional barriers are those that we have more control over, and they revolve around our perceptions of self-efficacy and other patient-related needs and preferences that may or may not align with the treatment itself.

CHAPTER 6

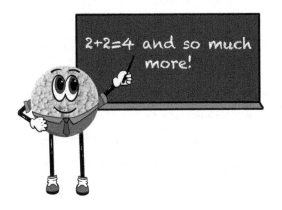

RICE CAKES AREN'T SO BAD (PUTTING IT ALL TOGETHER)

I was once giving a basic nutrition lecture, complete with the usual diet and lifestyle recommendations for heart disease, cancer, hypertension, and weight management. During the requisite Q&A period at the end of the lecture, a woman stood up and said, "I was recently diagnosed with cancer. I'm sixty, and I can honestly say that I have followed pretty much all of your recommendations for at least the past thirty years. I'm a runner; I eat an incredibly healthy diet and pride myself by staying up-to-date on the latest recommendations in the medical community. How can you promote all of the guidance in this lecture, when this can happen to someone like me?"

The entire audience, as if of one body, turned to me expectantly for an answer. I took a deep breath and gave my best answer to this common question: "I'm so sorry to hear about your diagnosis. This is a scary time, and I hear your frustration. But can I ask you to consider that perhaps your diagnosis might have come earlier in your life if you hadn't been so vigilant, that your personal regimen actually staved off your disease? And can I also ask you to consider that your outcome going forward is going to be way better because of how you've taken care of yourself in the past?"

The woman got out of her seat and came to hug me as tears ran down her cheeks. "Thank you," she said. "Nobody has ever said something so nice to me."

As I reflect back on this event, I can see many different elements of my practice come to life that contribute to the process of change. Did I learn how to respond to this woman in school or in later training? Not really. For me, the kind of answer I offered comes from life learnings—from my own life, from my counseling of others, and from my education about the psychological theories and modeling that I have found so supportive. The research I eventually did for this book in some ways confirmed some of the experience I had already attained, and other parts of this exploration served to add to, or enhance, what I felt I innately knew. It is the very definition of where art meets science!

My own journey has shown me how to put all of these pieces about the change process together into a bigger picture and view it as something that matters not only to me but to others as well. So, I'd like to show how all of this fits together—exactly what I promised in earlier chapters—the idea that acceptance, transformation, and healing take place most successfully when we consider and value the combination of emotions and established clinical confirmation. It works for all of us, patients and providers alike, and we can see this well-exhibited with the woman attending my lecture in the prior story.

The emotions this guest revealed were intense and justified. If you run through the litany of emotions she revealed, it reads almost verbatim like the list of emotions I experienced with my own diagnosis. We can hear her anger and frustration with me as the presenter, almost accusing me of putting forth inaccurate information about maintaining good health because she got sick anyway. We can understand her sadness for a former life of health and strength, one that she thought was fortified by her well-managed healthy regimen. We can also imagine her fear and sense of powerlessness as she struggles to imagine her future with this scary diagnosis, especially when she feels that her healthy regimen might not be as effective as she had hoped for and relied upon in the past. Remember that I, too, felt somewhat betrayed by my own body when diagnosed with celiac disease despite feeling healthy and without obvious symptoms. We see over and over again that, while the specifics of our lives differ, this kind of challenge to the status quo results in many common emotions.

There was also a glimpse into opportunities for acceptance and healing. I witnessed her grief about her diagnosis and about her feelings of powerlessness. You can imagine how much anger and frustration she had, thinking she "followed all the rules," yet was still met with a devastating and frightening diagnosis. No progress can be made without addressing this first. After witnessing her grief, I was able to help her reframe how she viewed her healthy behavior from "pointless" and not helpful in preventing disease to an understanding that her healthful outlook might have had a protective or, perhaps, curative role.

In response to her situation, I didn't ask her to "move on" or dissolve her grief before she was ready; the phrase "please consider" allows acceptance to occur with a pace that is more palatable to the patient. My answer to her question paved the way for additional possibilities for exploration; we can make sure we understand other motivations and fears through thoughtful, motivational interviewing and guided conversations. This was a perfect opportunity to address concrete and non-concrete barriers that might impede treatment, the kind of griever we are dealing with (out loud, practical, controlling, private), or information that might not have been offered by other healthcare providers. Any of these might adversely affect her attitude toward her disease and her ability to manage it.

This interaction was, admittedly, in a public setting, but I can imagine a private counseling session with this woman where we might explore and apply some of the more clinical prescriptions and applications.

- Remember those psychological models of behavior? Their guidelines would offer cues for directing her treatment based on how she perceives the benefits of adherence, how effective she feels in her own treatment, and how she views her interactions with her provider.
- I've led support groups over the years and, because of their helpful bond of shared experience, I'm a *big* fan. This would be an ideal intervention to recommend to this woman. Support groups play a role in filling the gaps that traditional treatment with doctors might be unable to focus on, such as extra

time for dealing with emotions or helping
with coping skills directed specifically at
one's particular diagnosis or condition.

- When we address understanding of an illness
  or a treatment, we must make sure that
  incorrect facts or missing information are
  not contributing to feelings of loss and grief.
  Did this woman have all the information
  she needed to get on a good path for healing? Did she have correct information about
  her diagnosis, or are there erroneous facts
  sticking in her head that were preventing
  forward motion? Keeping a patient-centered approach can uncover what "facts" or
  misconceptions might be holding a patient
  back in his/her recovery.

- Plus, I'd address what I call outlier situations,
  which are those that might take this woman
  out of her everyday activities and challenge
  the ways she has to treat her illness. Travel,
  entertainment, and social interaction are inte-
  gral parts of our lives, influencing our success
  with and acceptance of overall change. Those
  times when we are taken out of our normal
  routine are perfect opportunities for intentional and non-intentional barriers to crop

up—and uncovering and addressing them can be instrumental in improving emotions and increasing adherence.

These delicate situations do require keeping one thing in mind: don't allow personal experiences and opinions to get in the way when counseling. Yes, you can commiserate about a common disease state, but don't think that people always feel the same as you do. For example, I belong to the minority of people who "eat to live" rather than "live to eat." And I have no problem eating the exact same thing every day, although I do, of course, have many "favorite" foods and very much enjoy the social interaction associated with sharing meals with others. Because of this, a quote that never fails to make me smile is, "It's just food, you only rent it," but I have found that few people find it as funny or as appropriate as I do.

It sure was clear from this woman's reaction that some emotional doors opened for her that she previously thought were closed. Putting concepts and ideas like the ones we've explored into practice—that recurrent combination of the subjective and objective—made it possible for her to move a bit further in her healing from this devastating and overwhelming diagnosis. I saw that a similar process happened for this woman as it did for me when I experienced instant relief when my own doctor "witnessed" my grief.

We can now take what we learned about underlying, more measurable contributors to adherence and apply that knowledge to promote different approaches in practice. It seems clear that combining conversations about both emotions and clinical theory can bolster positive results. This approach takes into account the whole patient and helps everyone involved get to the nitty-gritty faster. Tailoring the experience of change to a person's individual needs can have quite an extensive impact on adherence, especially when you have theoretical support to rely on. Such personalization can't help but foster feelings of collaboration and comfort in voicing feelings and concerns. Patient satisfaction increases when this happens, and therefore so do quality measures that are evaluated by health-care organizations.

Here are some best practices for promoting adherence that come from combining subjective and scientific support:

Know your sources. This has to be one of my first discussions with any patient. I even focus on this myself as I work through the vast amounts of information that are available to us these days. What are resources that can give us the most confidence and how do we find them? A good first step is making sure our resources "have letters next to their names."

In other words, are there good education resources and/or peer supported information backing up your chosen source? Most of the time, adequately credentialed individuals know the importance of—*and use of*—good, supporting research as the basis for their recommendations. In the realm of social media, there are tons of message boards, blogs, and other online gathering places that offer advice and experience from quite an array of people. Some are published by laypeople, some by "wellness experts," and others by credentialed experts.

Laypeople are perfectly capable of many things. But, as a group, they do not have the training or education to know how to put out reliable and consistent education that the scientific community would approve of. And a lot of online information is undated, so one frequently has no idea whether the discussions are still relevant today or are a holdout from a few years ago, or even a decade ago.

I've often heard celiac patients say to me: "But so-and-so blog said I couldn't have anything with vinegar in it. That makes it so hard and restrictive, and I can't stay on my diet because I can't find anything safe to eat unless I buy it myself and carry it with me!" In actuality, staying away from vinegar was a many-years-old recommendation from a time before the celiac community knew that distilled products (including vinegar) do not contain gluten in their final form, no matter what grain was used in the formulation process. Vinegar is found in many foods, condiments especially, so once a patient is adequately educated by a properly credentialed person who knows current, accurate information, a whole new vista of safe and acceptable mustards, ketchups, and salad dressings is opened up.

Gone are the days of carrying a bottle of salad dressing in one's pocketbook or car glove compartment like I did! It is easy to imagine how knowing such a small fact as this can help a person adhere to a regimen both at home and while traveling, no matter what regimen is being followed. So, knowing where to reliably get this kind of information is paramount. And it's also easy to see that—as the behavioral models predicted—finding dependable resources can increase one's sense of efficacy in treating disease and managing change.

I recently found another frightening example of

how one should not take advice from unqualified individuals. On a Facebook message board for people with diabetes who are following a keto/intermittent fasting plan, someone wrote the following: "I just started intermittent fasting, and my last blood sugar reading was 59. Is that good?"

Since our bodies are programmed to convert carbohydrates into energy, and intermittent fasting and the Keto diet are highly restrictive in carbohydrate consumption, one's blood sugar on this diet can get pretty low as the body fights to find substitute energy sources for normal bodily functions. For the record, a blood sugar reading of 70 marks the level at which blood sugar must be raised on an urgent basis to prevent unconsciousness or even death. So, no, 59 is not good—it needs immediate attention! As an aside, not one of the members of this message board responded with this essential warning.

Great care must be taken when implementing new regimens, rather than relying upon the recommendation of anonymous voices with questionable education on an online message board. Instead, I highly recommend that someone who is trying to manage his/her diabetes consider an alternate diet consult with a diabetes educator or a doctor to make sure that any new regimen fits individual needs based on his/her combination of medical history and medications.

If you multiply these examples many times over in many different situations and with respect to many different disease states, you can see how important the "letters after a name" are to a patient who is navigating difficult life changes and new regimens.

Establish good understanding. When presenting an argument for adherence, a good knowledge base of accurate information is key. We cannot act in a responsible manner if we don't have or don't understand the facts needed to support our behavior. A clear, manageable body of information must be presented to us, at our individual level of understanding.

Oftentimes, we are presented with a complicated explanation or a solution that doesn't seem to fit into our everyday life. Not everyone reads at the same level or speaks English with the same proficiency. Thus, we need to have a good understanding of the audience and be prepared to find or supply appropriate explanations and documentation.

In my own practice, I make it a point to know where to find education materials at different reading levels and in different languages. A "teach back" approach for assessing comprehension is also effective, especially when conducted in a stress-free environment without pressure or threat of embarrassment.

Make sure the task at hand is not too complicated. One of my most important discoveries when counseling individuals is that science can sound like a foreign language to some people. I personally love science, but for some people, "it just doesn't compute." Factoring in cognitive development and meeting a patient at their own reading level are cornerstones of those behavioral theories. So, developing the ability to put science into layman's terms might be just as important as the science itself. My biggest successes in counseling patients happen when the patient says, "Wow, nobody ever explained it to me like that!"

Making sure a task is not too complicated also involves preparing for outlier events. In other words, we need to prepare, with good decision-making skills, for those occasions when we find ourselves in times or places that are not normal for us but where adherence is still important. It's common and, frankly, expected that success with adherence may suffer when we are away from home or on a different schedule.

For instance, I had two patients who were each overwhelmed by the details of the diagnoses they were accommodating when in difficult "outlier" situations. The first was a woman from one of my celiac support groups. She had unfortunately been hospitalized in ICU for an infection and eventually developed sepsis (an extremely serious overall infection of the blood). She was so focused on the medication (and its gluten content) being used to treat her life-threatening condition that she refused all treatment until the hospital pharmacist could confirm that no gluten-containing medications would be used. "I was almost dead for forty-eight hours while they figured things out, but I stayed gluten-free!" After this experience with this ICU patient, I developed a resource guide that helps with finding gluten-free drugs. I use it frequently with new patients when I try to address this kind of misguided decision-making in unusual circumstances.

I also got to know the second patient as a result of an interesting scenario where the path to adherence seemed overwhelming and complicated. After I had heard that one of my pediatric patients recently spent the night in the hospital, I investigated a bit and found out that this boy, recently diagnosed with celiac disease, went to a baseball game with his family during one of those incredibly hot and humid East Coast heat waves. The family only had a few bottles of water left, and everyone except the boy had drunk from those bottles after eating those yummy, baseball stadium soft pretzels. The boy had finished his own water and was understandably still thirsty because of the heat, but the mom, for some reason, was unable to purchase or provide a fresh bottle for him and would not let him drink from the other bottles that the family had shared. He wound up becoming dehydrated and spent the night in the hospital for observation and extra fluids. I was thankful to talk to the family after the boy was discharged, and we brainstormed about carrying personal water bottles and locating refilling stations, as well as the option of drinking soda in an emergency situation, even if soda was usually forbidden in their house. Talking more about the logistics of that day removed some of those overwhelming feelings and helped this family's future efforts to stay gluten-free when outside their home in challenging situations.

Making sure tasks are not too complicated also means finding good resources, easy explanations, and simpler tasks to mediate any temptation or possibility for nonadherence. Little sayings or mnemonics, such as my favorite "the trend is your friend," go a long way to help individuals stay interested and engaged, and they are applicable to many situations like weight loss and blood sugar readings. I still smile when I remember a young patient with diabetes who, upon seeing a month-long record of her blood sugars, exclaimed, "Look Mommy, the trend is my friend!" Another favorite example of how to simplify complicated instructions is the general guidance to the celiac community to treat gluten as "dirt" when dealing with cross-contamination issues. Simple instructions for washing with soap and water not only takes the gluten away, but makes for an easier and more understandable cleanup than most people realize.

Grow motivation by finding what makes an individual tick. Part of the PCC is to get inside the patient's head to understand what might cause success and failure. Wouldn't it be helpful to determine what induces anxiety, excitement, success, and failure in a particular individual?

A widely used technique for this is called motivational interviewing, or MI. MI attempts to "interview" an individual, pinpointing goals and optimal behaviors, as well as uncovering challenges and barriers that stand in the way of accomplishing these behaviors. This method takes into account that our actions and reactions are shaped by our history, influencing how we find support, choose doctors, relate to others, deal with authority, learn from mistakes, and deal with discomfort and adversity. MI teases out details that help us fit treatment to personality: what are our learning strengths, do we like to do our own research, or do we like to be fed information?

Because of the interactive nature of this conversation or "interview," individuals feel a part of the conversation and are better able to help uncover obstacles to their goals. Patients, it's important to actively seek out providers who regularly practice this important aspect of counseling. I was once inspired by a therapist who used the conversation starter "I'm curious," and I now use it in my own interview excavations. The phrase is a bit disarming and quite casual, and I have found using it usually opens the door to extra clues about what might work and what might not. Motivational interviewing, which underscores and values the infinite variety of human response, offers another approach to finding solutions regardless of personal situations or characteristics that prevent success. MI is flexible enough to meet the patient at their individual level of comprehension and readiness to change.

Support. Support from family, friends, and community is a big part of PCC. Studies have shown that individuals with little family support are less adherent to regimens, while individuals with more support at home are more adherent. Support can be practical, such as providing help to get to and from appointments or to fill prescriptions, or it can take the form of a teammate who provides encouragement or helps to maintain goals. Early focus on the kind or amount of support an individual already has can uncover needs and shortfalls that, when addressed, can help increase adherence.

For children with diabetes, it has been found that when a caregiver uses the "sharing" function on a glucose measuring device, such as a continuous glucose monitor, the correct usage of the device increases significantly and overall blood sugar levels are improved. The synergy of accountability and support from the caregiver is clearly a winning combination for young patients.

When I managed the celiac center, I saw firsthand how support groups were one of the best ways for my patients to gain comfort and encouragement, no matter where they were in their individual journeys. Some of the adult couples became socially active together, dining out and vacationing as a group. Some of the parents of celiac children developed their own "celiac-friendly" playgroups. And some adults and children became active in a local diabetes summer camp—what a great way to have your disease/regimen take a back seat to other, more pleasurable activities! I am one hundred percent convinced that the emotional impact of a positive support system is clearly reflected in an individual's sense of personal control and feelings of self-efficacy.

Support groups can also help us get perspective on our challenges. While we might think we have pulled the short straw by being forced into change, sometimes helpful input from others shows us that we are not alone and that others struggle too. My experience at a health fair when I ran the celiac center did just that!

The health fair was sponsored by FARE: Food Allergy Research and Education (formerly known as FAAN: the Food, Allergy and Anaphylaxis Network), an organization that supports individuals with food allergies and high-risk anaphylaxis reactions. While celiac disease is not an allergy per se, the gluten-free diet is often followed by individuals from this population, and education about any intolerance seemed to be a good fit for this health fair. Or so I thought.

All of the wind left my sails when a woman came up to my table and said, almost verbatim, "So, you think the gluten-free diet is hard? My son is allergic to corn, wheat, milk protein, and eggs, and has anaphylactic reactions to peanuts. Try living with that!" This woman, and her situation, quickly catapulted me out of my own agenda and into her world as she described what she was dealing with. Honestly, I was a bit dumbfounded and tongue-tied at the time and probably mumbled something trivial and ineffective. But this woman drove home how difficult her challenges were and how much she needed and valued the comprehensive, all-encompassing support this national support organization offered, instead of my solitary gluten-free table with its meager offerings! As a result, I became more appreciative than ever of support groups.

Make sure technology works for *rather than* against. Reminders on one's phone to take medication are a simple way to encourage adherence. Highly technical apps that are not intuitive and make the unsavvy user feel inhuman or neglected are counterproductive. Here, again, a technological tool is best and most effective when combined with the interactive relationship with the healthcare provider. A great example is telephonic counseling combined with text messages or automated reminders—a solution that I have seen enhance adherence.

Be willing to go at the patient's speed. Although it seems obvious, understanding the current emotional state and overall receptiveness is key to adherence. Anyone who has worked in ICU has seen a number of extreme, acute challenges that make the prospect of overall lifestyle changes pale in comparison. My memories of my time in ICU include a seventeen-year-old permanently paralyzed by an ATV accident, and a man whose private parts had been attacked by a flesh-eating bacteria. Who could propose dietary and lifestyle changes at that moment in these individuals' lives? Again, we have to be careful to pick and choose appropriate times for intervention.

Have a plan. Have an idea as to where your plan is going. Most patients and providers are more comfortable and find more success when regimens are precisely prescribed rather than vaguely developed over time. I remember when one of my sons, a high school senior in the middle of his semester of driver's education, asked me, "Mom, how do you know *how* to get to the place where you are going? How do you know what roads to take and what turns to make?" Very cute, but he unwittingly underscored the idea that there are many steps to take before you get to a goal. It is helpful for me to think of this example frequently, because it perfectly illustrates how someone new to a situation cannot be expected to innately know the "route" and must be taught or guided first. Forward-looking vision, knowledge, and preparation are all required to execute those steps, and we can do this with a thoughtful, well-constructed plan.

Don't be afraid to change course. Having this thoughtful, well-constructed plan is all well and good, but be fully prepared to examine and reevaluate both your process and your progress during any journey of change. Many situations, needs, and outcomes evolve over time. It's like when the best-laid plans to start insulin pump therapy are stymied by an allergy to the adhesive on the sensor. Or maybe a weight loss plan isn't working well for an individual in an inner city with minimal access to fresh fruits and vegetables. Sometimes a plan simply needs to be revisited or adjusted.

I never allow myself to forget my handling and treatment of my son's allergies when he was in elementary school; he had a chronic cough almost all of the time and had mild asthma attacks when he played soccer. It was assumed that he was experiencing seasonal allergies, so our pediatrician put him on a regimen of Claritin, we used an inhaler for exercise, and we thoroughly cleaned the forced air vents in our home. Some of his symptoms were reduced but never cleared up entirely. Years later, as an adult, my son told me that he had come to learn he is allergic to cats. Was my face red when I realized that our practice of allowing the family cat to sleep on his bed at night during his early years was probably the major contributor to his "seasonal" allergy problem! With 20/20 hindsight, the tipoff was that his symptoms never went away with his first "treatments," and that's when I should have reevaluated and found a new course to approach his problem.

Always be prepared to revisit your plan as well as rethink the assumptions that were made along the way.

Don't be too proud to make adjustments by consulting with established resources and expert opinions.

No cookie-cutter solution will work in the setting of change and adherence. The possible approaches mentioned earlier have influences that are both subjective and objective and are as varied and numerous as there are people. Use this list as a launching pad to add to or adjust as you navigate change.

ESSENTIAL
HIGHLIGHTS

- Objective and subjective input together provide many different approaches to manage change.

- There are many best practices that come from this combination. What best practices do you embrace now, or what might you adopt in the future?

CHAPTER 7

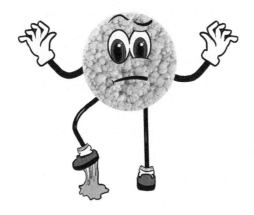

RICE CAKES DON'T ALWAYS WORK (GETTING UNSTUCK)

Back in my hospital days, I once was tasked with giving diabetes education to a woman who had just had her right foot amputated due to the complications of uncontrolled diabetes. Before I arrived in her room, I learned from some very frustrated nurses that this woman had developed quite the reputation of being generally uncooperative and verbally combative with everyone on the floor. She was clearly very angry and complained about everything, especially the diabetes "diet" that her doctor had prescribed for her stay. It was clear to me that, despite all the loss and change that accompanied the amputation, she was not yet in a place to implement any lifestyle changes that would aid in her healing or prevent further exacerbation of her disease.

After I introduced myself and we started to chat, she told me that she had been wrestling unsuccessfully with her diabetes treatment for a very long time and couldn't seem to implement the changes she knew were so important. She would try to "be good," as she put it, but then something would happen to cause her to backslide on any progress that had been made. She couldn't put her finger on any direct cause, but she kept saying, "I just feel so bad about myself."

As we explored various aspects of her life—her activities at home, her food intake, her medication regimen—she kept shaking her head, repeating, "It just doesn't work" or "I can't do that" over and over again. She seemed discouraged and paralyzed, incapable of seeing the benefits of any changes I proposed. After a while, I could see that she needed more than just the "best practices" I was offering.

While reading the preceding chapters, you may have said to yourself, "Well, things don't always work out quite so perfectly; not every situation gets wrapped up with such a pretty bow!" Yes, that is true. Not everyone wants to or is capable of retooling an entire life in the name of a prescribed lifestyle change. Nor does every situation resolve itself well, correctly, or according to schedule. And, as much as I would like it to, the objective and subjective combination approach doesn't always work, as I described in the previous story of the woman who had her foot amputated.

Sometimes we get stuck, paralyzed, and incapable of moving forward. We need to understand that this happens, to ourselves and to our patients. Of course, positive changes can still take place, even if those changes are not "normal" or are out-of-the-box. We have to allow space, time, and opportunity for when things don't go as planned and we need to get unstuck. Recognizing that things don't always go according to plan, I've included this chapter to add a few more approaches that will help explain what it means to be stuck and how we might guide people in this situation to help them move toward their full potential.

Sometimes we have overwhelming, disrupting feelings and self-criticism that make it hard to move forward. It's different from some of the other theories and approaches I've already described that concentrate on changing or supporting *behaviors* that get in the way of adherence in the face of change. Actually, our *minds* can defeat our efforts too!

Clinical psychologist Paul Gilbert, FBPsS, PhD, OBE, has put together a model that examines how we can first understand and regulate how our minds work and then develop compassion for ourselves when progress seems to have stalled. Let's explore this model because I believe that the woman described at the beginning of this chapter was experiencing some of the feelings Gilbert addresses: her forward motion had stalled, her health was at risk despite obvious and painful consequences, such as losing a foot.

EVOLUTIONARY VESTIGES IN OUR BRAINS

Gilbert's model, called compassion focused therapy, is all about how we deal with a "threat" to our existence and the actions we feel we have to take to relieve that threat. He describes how it all goes back to caveman times; we are hardwired to keep threats to our survival at bay to stay alive. Perceived hazards can, of course, be life-or-death situations that we must react to immediately, or in a more abstract sense, can take the form of other societal influences that challenge aspects of our lives that we hold dear: our health, families, livelihood, or general happiness. We can become anxious, depressed, or angry when confronted with such threats, and resort to flight-or-fight responses designed to rid us of the threat. The responses of combativeness (fight), evasion (flight), or indifference (freeze) were obviously quite useful in attacking, running away, or hiding from a saber-toothed tiger, for example, but they are, frankly, less efficient mechanisms for self-preservation today.

They are less efficient because sometimes they

make us overreact in the threat mode, creating an overly negative and extreme mindset that prevents us from reacting in more proactive and productive ways. So, our instinct to act against threat can sometimes work against us, keeping us from thinking as clearly as possible and hindering good decision-making processes—and adherence. For example, going back to my pre-diagnosis life in New Jersey, I was content with everything my life had to offer, but then the threat against everything comfortable and safe occurred with my celiac diagnosis, causing me to act out in unhealthy ways.

In the case of the woman at the beginning of this chapter, we can see the effect that the threat of diabetes had on her, as the "threat" of losing her foot left her mentally unable to weigh the benefits of adherence to her diabetes regimen against possible harm to her body. In this threatened state, she was unable to adhere to her diet and medication regimen at home, and she was combative and unreceptive when receiving medical advice in the hospital, despite how much she needed it.

Additionally, according to Gilbert, we humans also experience "drive," or the need to grow, produce, and experience new things. As positive and productive as this may sound, this innate need can also become exaggerated or distorted in our minds when things don't go well, stimulating a new "threat" experience. For example, if we set a goal (or have one set for us, such as a new diet or medication regimen) and then struggle or fail with it, we can berate ourselves to the extent that we actually feel threatened. In our minds, scolding ourselves can feel so unsafe, it's like confronting a saber-toothed tiger. It's common to chide ourselves with statements such as, "You think you are smart enough to handle this [change] but you really are stupid," or "You're sick because you didn't try hard enough." Such internal criticisms are examples of how drive can quickly deteriorate into a feeling of threat to our emotional or physical being. Then, the negative cascade of thoughts and actions begins all over again. The diabetic patient who lost her foot freely admitted that backsliding on her regimen threw her for a loop mentally, and her adherence suffered accordingly.

As a balance, according to Gilbert, we are also equipped with a way to combat the potentially destructive or inhibiting experiences of threat and drive by our ability to be soothed. This ability calms those threat and drive emotions, providing emotional balance. In previous chapters, we looked at how we can find help with soothing behavioral adjustments in the healthcare setting *outside* our bodies—such as support groups or participating in patient-centered conversations—but, as Gilbert describes, we can also self-soothe from *within*. This is known as self-compassion, an important tool to combat the negative and defeating emotions that can certainly get in the way of adherence to medication and dietary regimens.

EMPLOYING THE CONCEPT OF SELF-COMPASSION

When we criticize ourselves, we run the risk of escalating negativity and invoking the threat system. The threat system can inhibit rational thinking and prevent good decision-making. Criticism can come in many different forms and can happen in isolated events or as a constant barrage over time. Sometimes we call ourselves out or we scold ourselves with "should haves" or "could haves." Or we can come to the erroneous conclusion that one negative performance will translate into many or all future negative performances, further underscoring perceived inferiority in our minds. With this kind of threat undercurrent, it is understandable that our decision-making process can be negatively affected by this thought process.

I've certainly felt the threat to my own health and the discouraging feeling that comes with failing in my drive to succeed at living a gluten-free lifestyle. One of my earliest mistakes in learning how to live with a gluten-free diet was when I ordered a taco salad. This basic menu idea is that a salad, with whatever fixings you choose from the menu, is placed inside an enormous taco shell that serves as the bowl. I went to great lengths to explain to the waiter that I didn't want any croutons or any of the available salad dressings; I just wanted oil and balsamic vinegar, which was the go-to salad dressing in those beginning days when we didn't have much knowledge about ingredients. The waiter dutifully complied with each of my requests, and I proceeded to eat the salad ... and the bowl. The menu had described a "corn tortilla bowl," but I was still inexperienced enough back then to not know that many institutional or restaurant-grade corn products, like chips and tortillas, are actually a mix of corn and wheat.

Needless to say, I got very sick and felt very dumb, as if I might not ever learn what I needed to know in order to be successful in this new life. It seemed fair to rebuke myself back then, but I know now that this was an excellent learning experience certainly worthy of forgiving myself, with extremely profitable lessons for the future. I use this story frequently now, not to invoke a threat response in my patients, but to show how this kind of experience can, and probably will, happen to anybody and should be an occasion to show compassion toward ourselves for the hard work it takes to execute life changes.

According to Gilbert's compassion focused therapy, counseling in this situation is clear: have confidence and compassion for your decision-making capabilities. Yes, there is a threat, and that can be a bit paralyzing as we try to make constructive decisions during stressful times. But we are also smart, discerning people, capable of making our own decisions or enlisting the expertise of those we trust.

By talking with the patient I described at the beginning of this chapter about some of her past life experiences and how they influenced her decision-making processes now, we were able to uncover more about the emotions that colored her attitudes and actions related to her disease and amputation. Eventually, she was able to recognize these innate responses to the profound threat of her amputation and feel some compassion for her situation and her reactions. Because of our conversations, she gained an attitude that helped to temper some of the threatening feelings that had prevented her from working on monitoring her blood sugar, managing her carbohydrate intake, and increasing her activity level. I saw her a few more times before she left the hospital, and I believe she saw into herself and her behavior a bit more clearly by that time. Unfortunately, I was unable to follow up with this woman on an outpatient basis to gauge her progress, one of the disadvantages of working in a hospital.

There are many instances when we would do well to exercise compassionate behavior, both with ourselves and with others. As with the mother who withheld bottled water from her son at the baseball game because she thought the water might be contaminated with gluten, it is common for parents to be consumed with guilt and have a lack of confidence when faced with a significant diagnosis and change for their child. Most parents would say this is the very definition of a threat and a fight response! Oftentimes, caregivers summon up a protective reaction, even if they become negative, narrow, and inaccurate in their assessment and remedy of the situation, which is just what Gilbert predicted. It's apparent that, as a result of her own self-criticism, guilt, and self-doubt, this mother's reaction did become quite narrow in its focus when she decided to keep those gluten molecules away from her son, no matter the cost.

Or, consider the female ICU patient who was septic. She might have eased the threat she felt from potential gluten cross-contamination of her medication with some self-compassion for her very good knowledge base of celiac disease and the gluten-free diet with some compassionate self-talk: "Hey wait a minute. I don't want to die, and refusing much-needed medication on a short-term basis is not going to help my situation. The worst-case scenario of damaging my body by ingesting a few molecules of gluten now can be overcome by excellent adherence after I leave the hospital, and I can still regard myself as a responsible, healthy person after having experienced this. And, even if I made a mistake with this decision, I will forgive myself, view it all as a learning experience, and move on."

I love the idea of "self-compassion" as an antidote to perceived threat and self-criticism. Gilbert's glimpse into the mind wasn't really addressed in my formal education, but I wish it had been. Beyond the grief, the reframing, and the behavioral models addressed previously, compassion-based therapy uncovers our basic instincts for self-preservation and shows us how it is possible to make them work for us, not against us.

ANOTHER WAY TO GET UNSTUCK

A second and very pertinent theory for overcoming being stuck in the face of change or trauma is what is known as solution-focused therapy. Developed in the 1970s by psychotherapists Steve de Shazer, MSW, and Insoo Kim Berg, MSSW, solution-focused therapy is a process that focuses on solutions to problems rather than on the history or environment that created those problems. It instead promotes the idea that individuals come to a problem already possessing the knowledge and ability to form solutions and simply need help to recognize and harness the strengths and skills that are already inside of them.

I have a strong recollection of an episode I saw on a TV show many years ago. A woman was interviewed about how she was kidnapped, sexually assaulted, and left for dead by the side of the road. The details were horrific, and the woman was experiencing quite a bit of difficulty processing and recovering from fear and anxiety as a result of this traumatic experience. But instead of focusing on and trying to "cure" the fear and anxiety, the interviewer focused on something else. He asked her, "What were the things that you thought and did that ultimately resulted in your survival?"

With a few more pointed questions, he extracted several important behaviors that the woman unconsciously used to get through the situation: she used the same calm voice with her attacker that she used to de-escalate situations she had experienced with an abusive ex-husband; she knew from watching previous TV programs not to allow her attacker to take her to a second, isolated location; and she played dead when dumped in a ditch on the side of the road. In other words, even under the extreme stress of her attack, she tapped into prior knowledge and known inner strengths to come through the situation alive.

Solution-focused therapy capitalizes on this message. It says, "Look at what you brought to the situation—all your strengths, intelligence, resourcefulness, and experiences. You are a hero, not a victim. Now that you know how strong you are, you can use this power to overcome the trauma you are experiencing now *and* to channel this awareness of your inner strengths to help with future incidents or stressors." This model of therapy literally separates who we think we are from what happens to us, shifting the focus from adversity to what we want to achieve. Instead of looking at trauma as destructive and something to overcome, it builds us up and prepares us for the next time.

I believe the mom who withheld her son's water could have benefitted from this model of counseling as well. I bet if you asked her what she brought to the new situation to help her son and her family adopt a gluten-free diet in their lives, she'd recount an abundance of attributes: intelligence, flexibility, emotional strength, and the ability to withstand the pain of childbirth. The pointed questions and comments of solution-focused therapy can highlight these strengths and focus on the good decisions she has already been making for her son. Then the stage is set for incorporating these qualities during future stressful events. She's already the star of her own story!

The brothers who frequented the all-you-can-eat buffet also benefitted from elements of this model when I shifted the focus from how doctors were making them feel bad about their habits at the buffet to developing an outcome that worked for them. Clearly they were intelligent and had had successful careers earlier in life; my work with them helped to channel all of the talent that already existed into figuring out how to marry the convenience of the buffet line with managing their disease. Redirecting their feelings about who they were and all the life experience they brought to the situation helped them say to themselves, "I can do this!"

Everyone gets stuck at some point in their lives. Keep these forward-looking, compassionate tools handy when other tried-and-true models don't work or don't seem appropriate.

ESSENTIAL
HIGHLIGHTS

- Compassion-based therapy promotes an understanding of the fight-or-flight response in the face of life-altering change and uses that understanding to power a compassionate mindset for future healing.

- Solution-focused therapy uses the knowledge and strength that an individual innately brings to a stressful situation and redirects that energy to positive reaction and growth during future stressors.

CONCLUSION

I don't believe that the journey of change to adherence is ever finished. Adapting to a life-altering event is a lifelong process with many ups and downs along the way. Most people yearn for a preconceived view of life but may at some point find the need to acknowledge and address disappointments and challenges that are unexpected and unwelcome. Although we might be able to think of someone in our travels who seems to float through life unchallenged and unchanged, for the most part, we all share the basic human experience that life doesn't always turn out the way we'd like. The reality is that the looming possibility for change and adversity is ever-present for most people.

When we come to understand the place that inevitable and undesirable change holds in our lives, we are well on our way to getting to the ultimate goal of empowerment that I described at the beginning of this book. If we listen to and adopt the combined lessons of emotional awareness and impartial analysis, we will find a rewarding path to fuel recovery, healing, and growth.

Rather than accepting simple, sterile directives or cookie-cutter demands for compliance, the process of welcoming change and finding empowerment is actually a bigger idea, more than just "living to see another day." The fusion of the subjective and the objective presents enhanced options for us to view life-altering change, and to take new and improved command over our future behavior and responses.

Empowering behavior sometimes needs to be developed with education and counseling, but we have seen that we can start with what we already know about ourselves in order to get to our happily ever after. Changes to our lives highlight details about our overall beliefs, our sense of self, and specific skills and talents that exist independently from the change itself. I believe that without change, we might not really dig too deeply to evaluate and appreciate such inner strengths and capacities. It's an extreme version of making lemonade out of lemons when we become aware of exactly who we are and what we are made of.

At the time of my diagnosis, Dr. Rice Cakes surely did not have much experience with celiac disease or any confidence in my adherence to the gluten-free diet. However, his unsympathetic directive to "eat your rice cakes" unexpectedly lit a fire under me and made me realize that I really was competent and on a path to working things out.

- I became newly and happily aware of my own capacity for resilience and resourcefulness when I worked through the emotions related to grief and buy-in.

- My learnings about psychological theories and models pushed me further toward acceptance and healing than I ever expected possible at the time of my diagnosis. I found it encouraging and grounding to know there were data and theories to back up how I managed my feelings and experiences.

- I continue to use the lessons of compassion-based therapy and solution-focused therapy every day! These theories, in particular, help expand my awareness of myself and my reactions, and empower me toward acceptance on a daily basis.

The classic story in *Who Moved My Cheese* by Spencer Johnson, MD, depicts the evolution of change-related responses. It uses the metaphor of people and mice moving through a maze in order to find their ultimate goal of comfort and happiness, which is symbolized in the form of unlimited cheese. The lesson of the book is what happens to the characters when they discover that their "cheese" has been "moved" away from where they expected it to be, drastically affecting their prospects for ultimate happiness and the achievement of their goals. We are shown how each character brings to this situation emotions and behaviors that align well with the subjective and objective ideas put forth in this book. As we might expect, the characters' responses are colored by this internal input, giving some the confidence to accept and adapt positively to the moved cheese, while others were not able to accommodate the change and remained stymied in their future endeavors.

This story beautifully illustrates our mandate going forward. My own "cheese" has been moved several times. And coming to understand subjective reactions and clinical theories, like those put forth in *Eat Your Rice Cakes*, have certainly allowed me to heal and forge new directions when this kind of monumental shift happened along the way. I have found strength and determination to craft an existence that is filled with accomplishment and hope instead of failure and disappointment.

First, I healed myself. Grappling with my emotions and finding support and commiseration where I could when first diagnosed, I took my first steps toward finding acceptance in my new reality. As time went on, I applied what I knew about grief and the next step of "meaning" to my feelings and actions; this resulted in a healing mindset that ultimately opened up doors for me professionally, where I was able to help others who were experiencing similar life changes. Later in my professional life, psychological theories and models related to behavior change became happy confirmation for what I already knew: that our behavior has very deep roots in and is very definitely shaped by our history.

Thus, this subjective and objective combination was initially instrumental in my own healing, and it continues to resurface in all aspects of my life. Through the lens of this dual perspective, I can see that my diagnoses have changed me in the way I see and talk to myself and how I see and talk to others. Patients and providers are both participants in this emotional evolution, and my own ability to approach the topic from both perspectives has been invaluable when managing and integrating change.

More than ever, I embrace the power of reframing my undesirable thoughts and have found great success in sharing this healing concept in my work with patients. I find new strength in self-compassion and solution-focused exercises, both of which have helped me in my grief about celiac disease and unborn children. For sure, I've come to know great success in this mandate to fuse and synthesize, putting all of this together toward accepting changes and letting go of elements from the past.

In the end, I wanted to write a book about growth and empowerment, not passivity and ineffective deference to change. Whether we like it or not, life events and personal experiences will always crop up and change our plans and outlook. For me, the experience of my "Oreo Escapade" continues to resurface as I see similar reactions to change in others. And I'm happy to see that growth and empowerment are clearly part of these reactions. I have gained a greater understanding of and compassion for myself, and I rely on these sentiments each day to offer *and deliver* that same understanding and compassion to others.

As we contemplate how prescriptive ideas put forth in *Eat Your Rice Cakes* might integrate with how we manage alterations to life's plan, a good first step is to focus on our own thought processes and how influential they might be on behavior. Patients and providers can both participate and benefit from self-evaluating where they stand.

How do we regard the patient views of change? The provider views? Are we incorporating some of these patient-centered perspectives that lead to *adherence,* or are we still thinking that providers must force us to *comply* under their ultimate authority and control? Are we inviting collaboration into the mix? And are we applying those impactful and constructive learnings about cultural competence to our behavior?

Let's all strive to be on the same page about this as we pursue that mandate central to this book—to discover the stumbling blocks of change and find ways to accept and incorporate the change into life going forward. For me, it was the symbol of eating rice cakes to facilitate my healing, but each change and solution varies from person to person. Regrettably, clinicians don't always agree with each other or accept the same theories when it comes to how this process is managed. Remember the doctor who didn't like how I treated his homeless diabetes patient? Number one on *my* list is promoting a more collaborative mindset within the healthcare community and resolving the conflict between the concepts of compliance and adherence. I know that the best focus is on being flexible and finding what works so that outcomes continually improve over time, and I'm going to work on sharing and reinforcing this viewpoint.

These concepts are universal to most people, and the translation can be made to almost any human experience. Both patients and providers can apply to their present and future experiences these learnings about the human reaction to significant change. At the very least, one can use these ideas as conversation starters. At the most, we can hope for forward motion and healing in specific ways.

When I left my most recent job at the pharmaceutical company, I moved from New Jersey to Colorado, thinking I might retire. But instead, that move turned out to be part of an evolution in and of itself; I realized that I could see in front of me many new ways to apply my chosen profession and discovered in myself an interest in public health. After all, what is all of this for if not for the greater good? Chronic disease can feel bleak, and providers have to work hard to see that no patient falls between the cracks or is left unnecessarily vulnerable. And my ICU experience at the beginning of my career taught me one true thing: the stronger a patient is as they go *into* the ICU, the better chance s/he has of *leaving* the ICU alive. So, these days, I am focused on getting at-risk populations healthier in anticipation of future pandemics and challenges to our healthcare systems, knowing that the combination of subjective and objective approaches will be the centerpiece of my efforts.

One clear lesson Dr. Rice Cakes left with me is that we have a lot of work to do to fill in the spaces where compassionate care is lacking. If the objective and subjective combination detailed here is new to you, then assimilate it into your current practices and run with it. If you already espouse similar sentiments in your present life and career, please stay the course and teach others about it too. Either way, we have this amazing opportunity to share and implement this compassionate and effective mindset in our travels.

I can attest to an extraordinary level of satisfaction that advocating this viewpoint has brought to me personally and professionally, and I guarantee you will experience similar rewards. Have you ever purposefully articulated your own philosophy of patient care and education? That is a good way to examine where your thinking lies now and then to refine your outlook and forge new directions. Let us all thoughtfully grow and incorporate ideas of compassion, growth, and healing into this ever-changing world around us.

As of the writing of Eat Your Rice Cakes, *it is exactly twenty-five years since my celiac diagnosis and the "Oreo Escapade." I am content, no longer angry or defiant about my significant life changes. Family get-togethers are easily gluten-free, as we've had decades to gather and perfect many recipes—and we've even added a few vegetarians and vegans to the family mix along the way! I'm volunteering at my local community clinic, providing nutrition and diabetes education to underserved patients in my community. I'm also delving into the telehealth arena, because I see the advantages and enhancements that this platform offers the healthcare industry as growing exponentially over time.*

Writing this book has come with its own surprises of new healing and synthesis; I could not have imagined what an exciting, moving, and introspective adventure this has created for me! I thank every experience and person for their invaluable contribution to this life I lead, and for giving me the realization that change is not an isolated event to be rejected and condemned but is instead something that exists on life's continuum to be adopted and accepted.

Everything is integrated, not a struggle, and has become part of me. I have true gratitude for what I have now, for the meaning I have created so far in my life and in the lives of others, and for what is still to come.

Shut up? No way! I'm right here,
eating my rice cakes!

APPENDIX

RESOURCES FOR
CLINICAL THEORIES

HERE ARE INTERESTING ARTICLES and books that will help further your research about the formal psychological theories put forth in this book.

ARTICLES

Rosenstock's Health Belief Model, original paper published in 1974 by Irwin M. Rosenstock, PhD:

Rosenstock, Irwin M. "Historical Origins of the Health Belief Model." *Health Education Monographs* Vol. 2, Issue 4 (December 1974): 328–35.

The Theory of Planned Behavior, original paper:

Ajzen, I. "From Intentions to Actions: A Theory Of Planned Behavior." In J. Kuhl & J. Beckman (Eds.), *Action Control: From Cognition to Behavior* (Heidelberg: Springer, 1985), 11–39.

The Necessity-Concerns Framework, discussion on adherence within this theoretical framework:

Horne, Rob et al. "Understanding Patients' Adherence-Related Beliefs about Medicines Prescribed for Long-Term Conditions: A Meta-Analytic Review of the Necessity-Concerns Framework," *PLOS ONE* 8(12) (2013): e80633. https://doi.org/10.1371/journal.pone.0080633.

Information-Motivation-Strategy Model, discussion on intervention strategies related to this theoretical model:

Fisher, William A., Jeffrey D. Fisher, and Jennifer Harman. "The Information-Motivation-Behavioral Skills Model: A General Social Psychological Approach to Understanding And Promoting Health Behavior," *Social Psychological Foundations of Health and*

Illness 22 (2003): 82–106. https://doi.
org/10.1002/9780470753552.ch4.

Patient Centered Care Model, definition, benefits, and
examples provided by NEJM Catalyst:

NEJM Group. "What Is Patient-Centered
Care?" NEJM Catalyst. Last modified Jan. 1,
2017. https://catalyst.nejm.org/doi/full/10.1056/
CAT.17.0559.

Cultural Competency, definition and applications
provided by the CDC:

Centers for Disease Control and Prevention.
"Cultural Competence In Health and Human
Services," National Prevention Information
Network. Last modified Oct. 21, 2020. https://
npin.cdc.gov/pages/cultural-competence.

Saha, S., P.T. Korthuis, J.A. Cohn et al. "Primary
Care Provider Cultural Competence and Racial
Disparities in HIV Care and Outcomes." *Journal
of General Internal Medicine* 28
(2013): 622–629. https://doi.org/10.1007/
s11606-012-2298-8.

BOOKS

Kübler-Ross, Elizabeth, and David Kessler. *On Grief and Grieving: Finding the Meaning of Grief Through the Five Stages of Loss* (New York: Scribner, 2005).

Johnson, Spencer. *Who Moved My Cheese? An A-Mazing Way to Deal with Change in Your Work and in Your Life* (New York: Putnam, 1998).

Strayed, Cheryl. *Tiny Beautiful Things: Advice on Love and Life from Dear Sugar* (New York: Vintage Books, 2012).

Strayed, Cheryl. *Wild: From Lost to Found on the Pacific Crest Trail* (New York: Vintage Books, 2012).

NATIONAL SUPPORT ORGANIZATIONS AND CLINICAL RESOURCES

CELIAC DISEASE

National Celiac Association
20 Pickering St.
Needham, MA 02492
Boston Area: 617-262-5422
Toll Free: 1-888-4-CELIAC
Email: info@nationalceliac.org

Beyond Celiac
PO Box 544
Ambler, PA 19002-0544
Phone: 215-325-1306
Email: info@beyondceliac.org
Website: beyondceliac.org/

Celiac Disease Foundation
20350 Ventura Blvd., Suite 240
Woodland Hills, CA 91364
Phone: 818-716-1513
Email: cdf@celiac.org
Website: celiac.org

Gluten Intolerance Group (GIG)
31214 124th Ave. SE
Auburn, WA 98092
Phone: 253-833-6655
Email: customerservice@gluten.net
Website: gluten.net

CENTERS OF EXCELLENCE

The University of Chicago Celiac Disease Center
5841 S. Maryland Avenue, Mail Code 4069
Chicago IL 60637
Phone 773-702-7593
Website: cureceliacdisease.org

Colorado Center for Celiac Disease
Children's Hospital, Colorado Anschutz
Medical Campus
13123 East 16th Avenue
Aurora, CO 80045
Phone: 720-777-6669
Email: celiaccenter@childrenscolorado.org
Website: childrenscolorado.org

Celiac Center at Beth Israel
Deaconess Medical Center
330 Brookline Avenue
Boston, MA 02215
Phone: 617-667-1272
Website: bidmc.org/centers-and-departments/
digestive-disease-center/services-and-programs/
celiac-center

Celiac Disease Center at Columbia
University Medical Center
Harkness Pavilion
180 Fort Washington Avenue, Suite 936
New York, NY 10032
Phone (adult): 212-305-5590
Phone (pediatric): 212-305-5903
Website: celiacdiseasecenter.columbia.edu/

Celiac Center at Thomas Jefferson
University Hospital
132 South 10th Street
Philadelphia, PA 19107
Phone (Philadelphia location): 800-533-3669
Phone (Bala Cynwyd, PA location):
800-533-3669
Phone (Voorhees, NJ location): 800-533-3669

The Center for Celiac Research and Treatment
Allessio Fasano, MD, Director,
Center for Celiac Research
Yawkey Center for Outpatient Services at
Massachusetts General Hospital for Children
55 Fruit Street
Boston, MA 02114
Phone: 617-726-8705

OBESITY

Your Weight Matters
(awareness, education, advocacy and support)
4511 North Himes Avenue, Suite 250
Tampa, FL 33614
Phone: 800-717-3117
Fax: 813-873-7838
Email: info@yourweightmatters.org
Website: yourweightmatters.org

American Association of Clinical Endocrinology
Disease State Resources (for providers)
Website: pro.aace.com/disease-state-resources/
nutrition-andobesity

Obesity Action Coalition
(awareness, membership, advocacy,
education resources)
Website: obesityaction.org

Rethink Obesity (for providers)
(FAQ, education materials)
Website: rethinkobesity.com

Truth About Weight (for providers)
(resources, the science of weight loss)
Website: truthaboutweight.com

DIABETES

American Diabetes Association
(information about self-management and care)
Website: diabetes.org

National Diabetes Information Clearinghouse
(resources and education about self-care)
Website: Http://diabetes.niddk.nih.gov

Centers for Disease Control and Prevention
Diabetes Division
(education and research for both pre-diabetes
and diabetes)
Website: cdc.gov/diabetes

National Diabetes Education Program
(education about self-care and medication)
Website: ndep.nih.gov/

Joslin diabetes Center
(education and resources)
Website: joslin.org

Juvenile Diabetes Research Foundation
(awareness and education about type 1 diabetes)
Website: jdrf.org

HEART DISEASE

American Heart Association
(education, caregiver/educator support)
Website: heart.org

Centers for Disease Control and Prevention
(statistics, journal findings,
downloadable resources)
Website: cdc.gov/heartdisease

Healthy People 2020
(resources for prevention, detection and
treatment)
Website: healthypeople.gov/2020/
topics-objectives/topic/heart-disease-and-stroke

The National Coalition for Women
with Heart Disease
(advocacy for detection, diagnosis, and treatment of heart disease in women
Website: womenheart.org

ACKNOWLEDGMENTS

Many thanks go to my new friends in the literary world! To Donna Mazzitelli, The Word Heartiste, my editor from beginning to end, you honed my manuscript into something I never dreamed possible. And you did it with seasoned skill and much-needed diplomacy! To Lisa J. Shultz, a member of my local book club and author many times over, you were more than generous with your time and your recommendations that helped to get me started on my writing journey. And thanks to everyone who helped me at My Word Publishing: To Rich Wolf for his publishing expertise and to Victoria Wolf, who understood this book's layout and illustrations exactly how I pictured them!

To my beta readers (in no particular order): Abby Blaustein, MS, RD, CDCES; Lesley Pearl, PhD; and

Ted Brodheim. Interestingly, you all come from different decades in my history, and your contributions to my life and this book are priceless to me. Many thanks for your time and thoughtful input.

To my IT consultants—Daniel Masiello and Thomas Masiello: I could not do the technical parts of publishing this book without you! Thanks for your hard work and for your patience with my lack of computer and internet mastery.

To my patients: Heartfelt thanks for allowing me into your lives, for allowing me to help with your most challenging moments. Your trust in me, your encouragement, and inspiration have taught me lessons that will live on and help others for years to come.

To my advisors and colleagues: I count with gratitude every favor, every friendship, and your tireless support as my career has evolved.

To my family: We're in this together! All my love as we navigate our ups and downs.

And last but not least, to Dr. Rice Cakes: Thank you, first, for showing me who I am not. And then, thank you for showing me who I am.

ABOUT THE AUTHOR

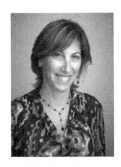

Margaret Weiss, RD, CDCES, is a dietitian and a diabetes care and education specialist. She graduated with a BA in psychology from William Smith College and completed her training in nutrition and dietetics at Saint Elizabeth University and the University of Medicine and Dentistry of New Jersey.

In addition to her own private practice, she has served in a number of healthcare roles in both hospital and ambulatory settings. She has appeared on the *CBS Evening News* with Jonathan LaPook and has been an invited speaker for grand rounds at several hospitals, national support organizations, the New

Jersey state dietetic association, and a New Jersey dietetic internship program. Her work has also been profiled in *Today's Dietitian* and several local New Jersey publications.

Formerly from the East Coast near New York City, she now lives in Colorado and enjoys trading in the stock market, hiking, and cross-country skiing.

Stay in touch with Margaret and find out about upcoming events at margaretweissrd.com.